Little, Brown Series in Clinical Pediatrics

Pediatric and Adolescent
Sports Medicine

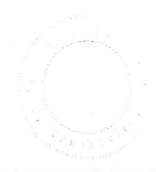

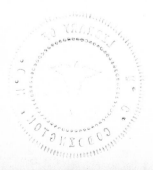

Pediatric and Adolescent Sports Medicine

Edited by

Lyle J. Micheli, M.D.

Instructor in Orthopaedic Surgery, Harvard
Medical School; Director, Division of Sports
Medicine, and Associate in Orthopaedic Surgery,
The Children's Hospital Medical Center,
Boston

Little, Brown and Company
Boston/Toronto

Library of Congress Catalog Card
No. 83-81536

ISBN 0-316-56949-6

Printed in the United States of America

HAL

This book is affectionately dedicated to my daughters, Amanda and Lisa, young sportswomen who have helped me to understand our new young athletes and dancers.

Contributing Authors

Robert C. Cantu, M.D.
Associate Chairman, Department of Surgery, and Director, Service of Sports Medicine, Emerson Hospital, Concord, Massachusetts

John B. Emans, M.D.
Instructor in Orthopaedic Surgery, Harvard Medical School; Associate in Orthopaedic Surgery, The Children's Hospital Medical Center, Boston

Douglas W. Jackson, M.D.
Director, Sports Medicine Clinic, Memorial Hospital Medical Center, Long Beach, California

Lana LaChabrier, M.D.
Consultant in Psychiatry, Division of Sports Medicine, The Children's Hospital Medical Center, Boston

John S. Leard, R.P.T., A.T.C.
Lecturer, Boston-Bouvé College of Human Development Professions, Northeastern University; Athletic Trainer/Physical Therapist, Northeastern University, Boston

Philip J. Mayer, M.D.
Assistant Professor of Orthopaedics, State University of New York at Stony Brook, Health Sciences Center School of Medicine; Director, Division of Pediatric Orthopaedics, and Head, Section of Scoliosis, The University Hospital at Stony Brook, Stony Brook, New York

Lyle J. Micheli, M.D.
Instructor in Orthopaedic Surgery, Harvard Medical School; Director, Division of Sports Medicine, and Associate in Orthopaedic Surgery, The Children's Hospital Medical Center, Boston

Gerald P. Reardon, M.D., F.R.C.S.(C)
Lecturer, Department of Surgery, Dalhousie University Faculty of Medicine; Orthopaedic Surgeon, Halifax Infirmary, Halifax, Nova Scotia

Nathan J. Smith, M.D.
Professor of Pediatrics and Orthopaedics (Sports Medicine), University of Washington School of Medicine, Seattle

Norman P. Spack, M.D.
Clinical Instructor in Pediatrics, Harvard Medical School; Associate in Medicine, The Children's Hospital Medical Center, Boston

William D. Stanish, M.D., F.R.C.S.(C)
Assistant Professor, Department of Surgery, Dalhousie University Faculty of Medicine; Orthopaedic Surgeon, Victoria General Hospital, Halifax, Nova Scotia

Linda K. Vaughan, Ph.D.

Professor and Chairman, Department of Physical Education and Athletics, Wellesley College, Wellesley; Visiting Research Psychologist, Exercise Physiology Division, United States Army Research Institute of Environmental Medicine, Natick, Massachusetts

John G. Yost, Jr., M.D.

Chief Resident, Orthopaedic Surgery, Lenox Hill Hospital, New York

Contents

Preface

Sports medicine is a new and rapidly developing area of interest in medicine and is, by its very nature, heterogeneous and multifaceted. It involves the study of the physiology and pathophysiology of sports and fitness participation and not only appropriately treats injuries resulting from sports participation, but also determines ways to prevent these injuries.

In the past, sports traumatology—the diagnosis and treatment of injuries resulting from sports participation—has received much more attention than other aspects of sports care, including the cardiovascular, nutritional, and psychological management of the athlete. Although appropriate and effective therapeutics is important in any area of medicine, perhaps particularly important in the care of athletes, the prevention of injuries and illnesses in those who take part in some form of sports and exercise is ultimately of equal or greater importance. The measures that will prevent the occurrence of heat injury or tennis elbow in the young tennis player should receive as high a priority as the effective management of either.

Ultimately, the most effective support for sports medicine as a unique discipline is its potential for the practice of true preventive medicine; that is, determining the host and environmental factors associated with the occurrence of a given sports injury or malady, and then taking steps to prevent these injuries or illnesses.

The need for both effective therapeutics and comprehensive preventive medicine is particularly important when dealing with young athletes who may risk special injury from sports training and participation. We now know that the child not only has a risk of special injury to the growth tissue from high energy trauma such as a fall, a twist, or a blow, but also may risk special injury from the repetitive microtrauma of sports training, such as throwing a baseball, vaulting in gymnastics, or merely running in a distance race.

These repetitive microtrauma injuries—the so-called overuse injuries—were once thought to be the particular bane of the unfit, adult weekend athlete and were believed to be rarely, if ever, encountered in children. We now know that overuse injuries can occur in anyone doing repeated movements—whether at work or at play—particularly if too much is done over too short a period of time without adequate preparation or conditioning of the body's tissues for this repeated pattern of stress.

In the past, children rarely performed repeated sports training movements to any great degree, since children's sports were relatively informal and often an extension of freeplay activity. Now we are seeing a dramatic increase in children's participation in sports, and hence in children's sports training. Not only are many more children participating in organized sports, but the intensity and duration of the sports training for these children is also increasing, sometimes with disasterous results. "Little League elbow," "swimmer's shoulder," and "gymnast's back," are a few of the "new" maladies being encountered in children. Another readily available example is the occurrence of stress or fatigue fractures in children, which was unheard of before the advent of organized sports training in this age group.

At present, pediatric and adolescent sports medicine is an area in which there are more questions than answers. Do children have a greater risk of physical injury from sports training than adults? Are the psychological stresses of organized sports competition for children excessive? Do children have special training needs for stretching, strengthening, or running, or are many of the techniques used by older athletes to prevent injury and improve performance unnecessary, or even dangerous, for children?

Unfortunately, many of the questions raised about children's sports are, as yet, unanswered. There has been very little systematic research into the training and physiology of athletically active children. The science of sports and exercise is a young one, and much of the work done has been on adults or elite athletes. In addition, although there are many experienced coaches for older athletes, at the high school, college, or elite level, there has been less attention given to systematic training of the grade school–level athlete. Experienced coaches of the child athlete are rare. Too often, coaches at this level are either totally inexperienced (volunteer coaches in community-based sports programs) or experienced in dealing with older athletes only. They are thus prepared to apply the same coaching methods to the child athlete, sometimes quite inappropriately. The active cooperation of physicians, physical therapists, athletic trainers, physical educators, coaches, and concerned parents is required to answer many of these questions and to improve the safety of sports participation by children.

The goals of any sports program should include enjoyment by the participant, enhancement of health and fitness through this participation, and the avoidance of injury. This is particularly important at the child's level, where an unenjoyable or stressful experience with sports or an unnecessary injury may have an adverse effect on physical activity and health for the rest of the child's life.

L. J. M.

Acknowledgments

I am pleased to acknowledge the generous help and patience of my fellow contributors to this work, without whose effort this book would certainly not have been possible. I am also pleased to acknowledge the help and encouragement of my colleagues and associates in the Sports Medicine Division of The Children's Hospital Medical Center. I am especially indebted to Ms. Daria Christensen, Lisa Hammond, and Katherine Adams for their help in the preparation of this work.

Pediatric and Adolescent Sports Medicine

NOTICE

The indications and dosages of all drugs in this book have been recommended in the medical literature and conform to the practices of the general medical community. The medications described do not necessarily have specific approval by the Food and Drug Administration for use in the diseases and dosages for which they are recommended. The package insert for each drug should be consulted for use and dosage as approved by the FDA. Because standards for usage change, it is advisable to keep abreast of revised recommendations, particularly those concerning new drugs.

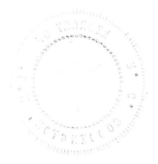

1. Sports Injuries in the Young Athlete: Questions and Controversies

Lyle J. Micheli

Organized sports competitions are becoming more and more common among Americans of all ages and at all levels of competence. The role that such competitions should play in both school and recreational activities for children has been a source of considerable controversy in recent years. The potential for serious physical or psychological injury has been suggested, and the relative risk of injury in organized sports versus free-play activities is actively debated. There are three areas of major concern: whether children are exposed to excessive emotional stress by participating in organized sports; whether children can undergo the physiologic stress of vigorous organized sports training and conditioning; and finally, whether the risk of serious injury to these children is increased because of their participation in these organized sports. For good or ill, though, the trend noted above seems irreversible.

A number of factors contribute heavily to the increasingly organized character of children's sports. The need to organize the use of limited recreational facilities, the progressive loss of open space and vacant lots in many cities and suburbs, and the decrease in spontaneous neighborhood activities are all involved. The proponents of organized sports for children argue that this organization benefits the child in a number of ways. The access to trained coaches improves the techniques of play at an early age and results in increasingly skilled participation later. The development of leagues, playoffs, uniforms, etc., increases enjoyment and helps maintain interest. Finally, properly supervised games have a lower risk of injury than free play. It is noted in the by-laws of the Pop Warner Junior Football League Association, which sponsors community-based football for 10 to 14-year-olds, that the specific objectives of the league are "to familiarize all boys with the fundamentals of football and to provide opportunity to play the game in a supervised, organized, and safe manner" [8].

The importance of play activity in the physical and emotional development of the child is well documented. Piaget has noted the close relationship between the development of motor skills and cognitive function [14]. Bauer, in his presidential address to the American Ortho-Psychiatric Association in 1972, cited peer play activities as one of the four key integrative systems "which gives pattern and meaning to the basic personality of the individual and to the society in which he lives" [3].

The transformation of play activity into sport activity appears to

1

have cultural determinants. Luschen defines sport as a "rational play-ful activity or interaction which is extrinsically rewarded. The more it is rewarded, the more it tends to be work: the less, the more it tends to be play" [11]. He hypothesizes that the main functions of sport are pattern maintenance and integration of the individual into society, and he cites studies of the process of socialization in which the exposure of children to competitive sports caused these children to become more achievement-oriented. The earlier this exposure occurred, the more achievement-motivated they became. Piaget has also noted the socialization function of organized games for the older child [14]. Schafer observed that the American sports subculture is inherently conservative, and that participation in sport probably leads more to acculturation into the established values of society than to any process of "character building" or to the development of independence [21].

PSYCHOLOGICAL STRESS

That participation in traditional games and sports, generally organized and directed by children themselves, is a valuable and healthy mechanism of acculturation is not seriously doubted by anyone. However, the relatively recent development in North America of vigorous, structured organized sports for the preadolescent child is a quite different phenomenon, and, as mentioned above, the benefits of this development have been questioned by many observers [11].

Parsons has argued that the young child is not emotionally mature enough to handle the psychological stress of league and tournament competition [13]. Similarly, Sayre has called for a ban on competitive sports involving preadolescent children because of the long term harm done to both the successful and unsuccessful child competitors [19].

Conversely, proponents of organized sports for children claim enhanced self-confidence and maturity for young competitors, and cite evidence that the emotional and mental status of these children was not significantly affected in any negative way by the competition, since tension, when evident, was short-lived. Early studies of the emotional impact of organized sports on children attempted to use physiologic parameters, such as changes in pulse, blood pressure, and serum catecholamines, to determine stress [16]. These studies, too, showed little negative effect. One such study, however, did find that one-third of the boys participating in Little League contests were too excited after the games to eat normally [24].

More recently, investigators have begun to evaluate the psychological and social effects of competition on children and the specific factors associated with organized sports stress in children using psychological testing procedures. Scanlan, using the Sports Competition Anxiety Test, found that such factors as the child's competitive and basal anxiety states, level of self-esteem, and expectation of self and team performance were significantly related to the stress experienced immediately before and after the game competition [20]. Other determinants of comparative stress were the amount of fun experienced during the game, parental and coach attitudes, and the perceived importance of winning the game to the coach.

Smith et al. at the University of Washington have been most interested in assessing the impact of the adult coaches on young players. Studying organized youth baseball and basketball, they found that children coached by personnel utilizing reinforcement and positive feedback techniques demonstrated enhanced self-esteem over the course of a single athletic season when compared to children in a coaching environment characterized by condescension and negative feedback [25].

To date, what few studies have been done on the psychological impact of organized sports on children have been short-term. They have generally dealt with a single competitive event or, at most, the duration of a single athletic season. Long-term studies of the psychological impact of organized sports competition of children are needed, but such studies are very difficult to do. The simple truth seems to be that whether or not an organized sport activity for children is beneficial depends on the structure of the particular sport and the quality of the adult leadership involved in the sport. A major cause of continuing concern and careful assessment of psychological stress in children's sports is that we have a situation in which our most susceptible athletes are often being handled by our least trained coaches.

In addition to the effect that the attitudes and behavior of the coaching staff has upon children, there is no doubt that the attitudes and responses demonstrated by collegiate and professional athletes also have a significant impact upon younger athletes. Unfortunately, the example set by these older sports participants, and even sports heroes, can often be far from exemplary. The emphasis put upon winning at any cost, the frequent glorification of violent behavior and fighting in such sports as hockey, baseball, and even basketball, and the not infrequent occurrence of overtly unsportsmanlike behavior often have a detrimental impact on both the volunteer coaching personnel and the participants at these younger levels. Martin Rublonski's *Lords of Locker-room: The American Way of Coaching and its Effect on Youth* [15] and Gary Shaw's *Meat on the Hoof* [22] vividly describe these bigtime coaching techniques and the environment they create.

Fortunately, there are numerous examples of organized sports systems, both here and abroad, where the competitive aspects of the game appear to be kept in perspective. Here the enjoyment of the participants is the primary objective. The sports clubs of Europe with their emphasis on competition at all levels of ability are mirrored in this country by such sports as gymnastics, rugby, and soccer, where participation and enjoyment are valued equally with winning.

It is beyond question that properly organized athletic programs for younger children can be highly enjoyable. Unfortunately, poor leadership and the emotional involvement of coaches and parents seeking vicarious gratification can turn organized children's sports into a charade of true sportsmanship. Too often, the adult participants place undue emotional stress upon young athletes without significantly improving either their playing techniques or their enjoyment of the game.

PHYSIOLOGIC STRESS

Despite the dramatic increase in organized sports for young children that has taken place over the past 15 years in this country, there is a scarcity of data regarding the effects of systematic training on cardiorespiratory or musculoskeletal fitness in children. In sports such as Little League baseball and Pop Warner football, of course, there is little sustained physiologic stress demanded of these children, and the fitness benefits of such sports are probably minimal. With the growing numbers of children participating in endurance sports such as swimming, distance running, and soccer, however, questions have been raised about the safety of exposing children to high levels of aerobic training stress, echoing the traditional concerns that children's (and women's) hearts are not "strong" enough for such sports. However, scarce though the data may be, what there is is reassuring.

The vigorous training and the physical stress of some organized sports do not appear to adversely affect the growth and development of children. Moderate physical training may augment growth. Astrand et al. observed that Swedish girls undergoing several years of vigorous training suffered no deleterious effects and actually appeared to be ahead of their age group developmentally [2]. Ekblom studied young boys undergoing vigorous physical activity and noted decreased body fat, increased lean body mass, and increased height, as well as a moderate increase in maximal oxygen uptake, when compared to those without extra training [7].

On the other end of the scale, lack of muscle use in an extremity, as in poliomyelitis, results in a relative lack of longitudinal and circumferential growth of the extremity [10]. It can be concluded that a certain amount of physical activity is not only beneficial, but also necessary to normal growth and development. No studies have yet shown that excessive physical activity and athletic training are harmful to the growing child, although it is probable that the necessary amount of physical activity for normal growth and development in children may be readily attained by free-play activities.

While some investigations of children involved in endurance sports such as running or swimming suggest that these young athletes do not demonstrate a significant increase in aerobic fitness, as measured by change in maximal oxygen uptake, as adults do [1, 5, 17], other studies have shown that the child is capable of a respons to endurance exercise similar to that seen in adults when compared to age group controls [6, 27]. When maximal oxygen uptake values are corrected for lean body mass, children appear capable of obtaining levels of cardiovascular fitness comparable to the most highly trained adults.

In the past several years, children have safely completed the marathon distance of 26 miles 285 yards in under 4 hours. Thus, if proper techniques of athletic training and conditioning are employed, with slow progressive increase in cardiovascular stress, children appear able to safely perform vigorous endurance training without difficulty. Whether they can do so without an increased risk of long-term musculoskeletal problems, however, still remains to be seen.

INJURIES

The possibility of increased susceptibility to injury, and especially musculoskeletal injury, in organized sports is the third area of concern and, again, remains a very controversial subject. There is evidence that the growing bones and joints of a child are more susceptible to certain types of mechanical injury than those of the adult, both because of the presence of growth cartilage, and the process of growth itself.

Growth cartilage is present at the growth plate, articular cartilage, and sites of major muscle-tendon insertion—the apophyses—in the child. The growth plate and articular surface of the child are more susceptible to shear and impact injury, while the presence of growth cartilage at the tendon insertions increases the chance of avulsion from the bone, particularly if the child is growing rapidly and these structures are further tractioned by the growth of the bones they span [12] (Figure 1-1). In a noncontact sport, where high-velocity trauma is not likely, the recurrent microtrauma of repetitive training, as in throwing practice, gymnastic practice, or distance running, can injure these tissues.

Excess

In certain circumstances, the organization of sports for children may increase the possibility of over-training. "Little league elbow," for instance, is not seen in free-play situations. In some sports—gridiron football, rugby, hockey, and soccer—the risk of injury, especially irreversible injury to the growth plate of the bone from high-impact trauma, may be greater when the players train seriously and play intensely. The young runner may be hurt by training too hard. The young football lineman, because of his training, may be playing too hard.

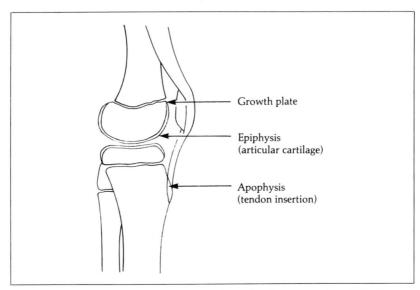

Growth plate

Epiphysis
(articular cartilage)

Apophysis
(tendon insertion)

Figure 1-1. Growth cartilage is present at three sites in the growing child: the growth plate, epiphysis, and apophyseal sites of muscle-tendon insertion. Each site is a potential site of injury in the child from single impact macrotrauma or repetitive microtrauma.

Fortunately, there is some evidence that the preadolescent athlete, even when engaged in organized contact sports, runs significantly less risk of injury than his counterpart at the high school or college level. Roser and Closen reviewed the incidence of injury in the Seattle Junior Football League for a two-year period. They found a 2.3 percent rate of injury among these young players and observed that few of these injuries were serious [18]. Godshall reviewed the records of the Pop Warner football programs in a Pennsylvania league in which 1,700 boys participated on various teams during a 12-year period. He found few major injuries. It was further cited by Pop Warner officials that there has not been a single fatality in 43 years of play.

More recently, studies by Sullivan et al. found an overall rate of injury in Oklahoma youth soccer of 2.6 per 1,000, with children under 10 years sustaining less than 1 injury per 1,000, while those of secondary school age were injured at a rate of 7.7 per 100 participants [26]. A similar relation was noted by Zaricznyj, with an injury rate of 3 per 100 at the elementary level, 7 per 100 for junior high school, and 11 per 100 at the high school level [28]. Despite the relatively low rates of injury recorded in some of these studies, however, some observers feel that the rate of injury in children's sports is increasing [9, 23]. They cite improper or nonexistent training techniques, poor coaching, and inadequate triage systems.

In the more traditional sports medicine setting, the injured athlete presented himself to the team doctor, often at the direction of, or at least with the approval of, the coach. If the team was fortunate enough to have an athletic trainer, the athlete may have had an initial assessment by the trainer before seeing the "Doc." The team doctor's primary role was to confirm the diagnosis, estimate the severity of the injury, and, most importantly, prognosticate return to action, in conjunction with formulating an appropriate treatment and rehabilitation program. In the design of a particular rehabilitation program for an athlete in a particular sport, the team doctor could usually count heavily on the resources of coach and trainer for supervision and progression.

Not so with the child athlete. Despite the fact that one of the prime reasons cited for the initiation of organized children's sports has been to decrease the chance of injury by proper supervision and the teaching of safe playing techniques, little if any attention has been directed to teaching these adult supervisors and coaches current concepts of safe athletic training or the preventive aspects of sports medicine. Even when these sports are a part of school physical education programs, medical supervision is usually fragmentary [4]. Although most states require physicians or emergency technicians to be in attendance at high school football games, this is not so for junior high school or grade school sports. In most of these school sports situations, coaches are volunteers from the faculty receiving supplementary income for their coaching time. Knowledge of the coached sport is variable and knowledge of proper conditioning and training techniques is often nonexistent. Medical coverage on-site may be the responsibility of the school nurse—who is often ill-equipped to assess or provide first aid for sports injuries, and the triage system often consists of a parent being called to drive the injured athlete to the family physician, pediatrician, or emergency room. The extent of this problem is reflected in a recent study by Zaricznyj et al., which suggested that school physical education classes produced almost twice the rate of injury of school sports in this age group [28]. However, the majority of sports activities in this age group occurs in organized community sports programs, not in the schools. This trend will doubtless increase in the next decade, as school programs face increased fiscal restraints. Sports programs, particularly in the lower schools, are usually the first casualties of cutbacks.

In community-based sports, physicians must assume increased responsibility for the initial assessment and triage of injuries, as well as their subsequent management and rehabilitation, and the appropriateness of training techniques. Finally, physicians must give good guidelines for returning to play.

REFERENCES

1. Astrand, P-O. Experimental studies of physical working capacity in relation to sex and age. Copenhagen, Denmark: Munksgood, 1952.

2. Astrand, P-O., et al.   Girl swimmers. *Acta Physiol. Scand.* [Suppl.] 147:3, 1963.
3. Bowel, E. M.   K.I.S.S. and kids: A mandate for prevention. *Am. J. Orthopsychiatry* 42:556, 1972.
4. Bowers, K. D.   Young athletes enduring alarming treatment delays. *Physiol. Sports Med.* 4:57, 1976.
5. Daniels, J., and Oldridge, N.   Changes in oxygen consumption of young boys during growth and running training. *Med. Sci. Sports* 3:161. 1971.
6. Ekblom, B.   Effect of physical training on adolescent boys. *J. Appl. Physiol.* 27:350–355, 1969.
7. Ekblom, B.   Physical training in normal boys in adolescence *Acta Paediatr. Scand. Suppl.* 217:60, 1971.
8. Godshall, R. W.   Junior League Football: risks vs benefits. *J. Sports Med.* 3 (4):139, 1975.
9. Goldberg, B., et al.   Children's sports injuries: Are they avoidable? *Physiol. Sports Med.* 7:93, 1979.
10. Green, W. T., and Anderson, M.   The problem of unequal leg lengths. *Pediatr. Clin. North Am.* 2:1137, 1955.
11. Luschen, G.   The interdependence of sport and culture. *Int. Rev. Sports Psychol.:* 16:27, 1967.
12. Micheli, L.   Sports Injuries in the Child and Adolescent. In R. H. Strauss (Ed.), *Sports Medicine and Physiology.* Philadelphia: Saunders, 1979.
13. Parsons, T.   Toward a healthy maturity. *J. Health Hum. Behav.* 1:163, 1960.
14. Piaget, J.   *The Psychology of the Child.* New York: Basic Books, 1969.
15. Rablovsky, M.   *Lords of the Locker Room: The American Way of Coaching and Its Effect on Youth.* New York: Peter H. Wyden, 1974.
16. Rarick, G. L.   Competitive sports for young boys: controversial issues. *Med. Sci. Sports* 1:181, 1969.
17. Robinson, S.   Experimental studies of fitness in relation to age, *Arbeitphysical* 10:251, 1939.
18. Roser, L. A., and Clauson, D. K.   Football injuries in the very young athlete. *Clin. Orthop.* 69:212, 1970.
19. Sayre, B. M.   The need to ban competitive sports involving pre-adolescent kids. *Pediatrics* 55:564, 1975.
20. Scanlon, T. K., and Ragan, J. T.   Achievement motivation and competition: perceptions and responses. *Med. Sci. Sports* 10:276, 1978.
21. Schafer, W. E.   Sport and youth counterculture: contrasting socialization themes. Presented at a conference on Sports and Social Deviancy. State University of New York, Brockport, December 10, 1971.
22. Shaw, G.   *Meat on the Hoof.* New York: St. Martin's, 1972.
23. Silverstein, B. M.   Injuries in youth league football. *Physiol. Sports Med.* 7:105, 1979.
24. Skubic, E.   Emotional responses of boys to little league and middle league competitive baseball. *Res. Q. Am. Assoc. Health Phys. Educ.* 27:97, 1956.
25. Smith, R. E., Smoll, F. L., and Curtis, B.   Coach effectiveness training: a cognitive-behavioral approach to enhancing relationship skills in youth sport coaches. *J. Sport Psychol.* 1:59, 1979.
26. Sullivan, J. A., et al.   evaluation of injuries in youth soccer. *Am. J. Sports Med.* 8:325, 1980.
27. Vaccaro, P., and Clarke, D. H.   Cardiorespiratory alternatives in 9- to 11-year-old children following a season of competitive swimming. *Med. Sci. Sports* 10:204, 1978.
28. Zaricznyj, B., et al.   Sports-related injuries in school-aged children. *Am. J. Sports Med.* 8:318, 1980.

2. Emergencies in Children's Sports
William D. Stanish and Gerald P. Reardon

There is nothing quite as frightening or disturbing for the sport enthusiast and those involved in sports medicine as the suspense and concern that surround an injured child athlete. The scene at such emergencies seldom varies, with medical personnel and bystanders rushing to the victim in anticipation of treating an injured ankle or sprained elbow. Suppose, however, they find the athlete lying in a moribund state, acutely apneic with a severe head injury, or suffering with respiratory embarrassment as a consequence of a tension pneumothorax?

Such distinct and dramatic injuries require immediate and skilled lifesaving maneuvers. Improper first aid treatment, tardy transport to a tertiary care hospital, or, more basically, unsound triage by the medical doctor at the scene of the injury, may cause unnecessary and tragic sequelae. The purpose of this chapter is to offer information on types of injuries and situations that are considered emergencies in children's sports and to describe the appropriate medical response.

HEAD INJURIES
Head injuries of varying severity are common in sports involving heavy physical contact, such as football and ice hockey, but are also seen in many other less physical activities.

Trauma to the head ranges from small lacerations that can be treated adequately at the scene, to an expanding intracranial hematoma with unconsciousness that will require specialized neurosurgical care.

In assessing any head injury, there are certain guidelines that should be followed. The history of how the injury occurred is vital, as is a report of the patient's level of consciousness following the accident, since a decreasing level of consciousness may indicate intracranial pathology such as a blood clot.

History-taking and physical examination repeated at frequent intervals are of utmost importance in diagnosing serious head injuries, as ancillary aids are few. Skull x-rays should always be done to demonstrate the presence or absence of a fracture. Sometimes special tangential views are necessary to illustrate depressed fragments. Computerized axial tomography (CAT) scans are invaluable in demonstrating intracranial hematomas. It should be noted, though, that a shift of the midline at the time of the initial examination may be the only abnormality present to indicate a hematoma. Since the advent of computerized axial tomography, arteriography is not usually necessary following acute trauma to delineate intracranial pathology. Lumbar puncture has no place in the early investigation of head injuries. It is a difficult procedure in the restless patient, and the presence or absence of blood in the cerebral spinal fluid yields no indication of the severity of the injury. If intracranial pressure is increased, the lumbar puncture may expose the patient to an added risk with possible catastrophic sequelae.

It is not necessary to keep head-injured patients dehydrated as was once the practice, but care must be taken not to overload the patient as this can aggravate cerebral edema and be a menace should nausea occur. If it is going to be some time before the injured youngster can arrive at a treating hospital, then administration of a 20 percent mannitol solution in a dose of 1.5 to 2.0 gm/kg is recommended as a temporary measure to decrease brain swelling and, thus, lower intracranial pressure. This is particularly vital in an injured athlete whose level of consciousness is decreasing with the worsening of his neurological function. If mannitol is unavailable, then 50 percent glucose may be substituted. However, these agents should only be used to buy time in a patient with a suspected surgical lesion with increasing intracranial pressure. Their routine use in patients with head injuries is to be strongly condemned.

Intravenous dexamethasone also is effective in reducing cerebral edema; however, its action is not apparent for upwards of 12 hours following administration. This makes its use somewhat impractical unless for some obscure reason transfer to a neurosurgical unit is delayed. Although the dexamethasone is really not very effective as acute therapy in contrast to mannitol, its use has been continued. The dose employed is usually a 10-mg intravenous bolus followed by 4 mg every 6 hours.

Antibiotics are only required for treatment of compound skull wounds. Ampicillin is usually the drug of choice.

If a child suffers a post-traumatic seizure, Valium is usually successful in terminating the episode. There is some controversy as to whether the child should be placed on long-term anticonvulsant medication.

INITIAL ASSESSMENT AND TREATMENT

As with any type of major trauma, initial attention should be focused on maintaining a patent airway. An unintubated child should be transported in a semiprone position to protect the airway and avoid aspiration. Vomiting is often seen following even minor head injuries and in itself is not a major cause for alarm, but the dreaded complication of aspiration is best treated by prevention.

Gross external bleeding should next be controlled. It must be remembered that although a great deal of blood can be lost through extensive scalp lacerations, hypovolemic shock is rarely due to head injury alone. Certainly in the absence of visible scalp bleeding, the patient in shock following head injury must be carefully evaluated for other hidden injuries, such as to the chest or abdomen. This is particularly true for the young athlete who has sustained extreme violence, such as being thrown from a horse during equestrian activities.

Following cardiopulmonary stabilization, assessment of the cranial injury can take place. A mini-neurological exam is briefly performed, and this should include evaluation of vital signs, assessment of the level of consciousness, examination of the pupils, presence of abnormal plantar reflexes, and evaluation of any weakness of one side of the body.

The keys to observing a child with an acute head injury are the repeated assessment of neurological function and the taking of vital signs at regular intervals. Following initial evaluation, further management depends on the answers to three questions:

1. Is there a decreasing level of consciousness?
2. Is there evidence of increased intracranial pressure such as bradycardia and high systolic blood pressure?
3. Are there any localizing signs—one-sided weakness, a dilated pupil on one side, or an extensor plantar response?

If the answers are positive to all questions, this indicates an acute emergency and neurological intervention is required. If all answers are negative, as they are in the vast majority of head injuries, these patients must continue to be observed closely. If there is any clinical evidence that the young athlete is not completely normal in terms of mentation and clinical signs, then he or she must not be returned to the athletic contest.

In summary, *the most important factor to observe in the head-injured young athlete is the level of consciousness.* Repeated assessment of the changing character of a young patient's clinical condition cannot be overemphasized.

Scalp Lacerations

Lacerations can be quite minor, requiring only a few sutures or, on the other hand, can be very extensive with major blood loss. All lacerations should be adequately cleansed and debrided. If properly equipped, then the attending medical person should carry out these procedures at the athletic contest, but the wound should not be explored for hidden foreign bodies and for underlying fractures. Quite clearly, this more extensive treatment should be carried out in a hospital setting. Lacerations longer than approximately 3 cm should have the galea closed as well as the skin. Tetanus prophylaxis should, of course, be administered if indicated.

SKULL FRACTURES

Any skull fracture, no matter how insignificant on x-ray appearance, should be assessed with some caution. The presence of a fracture indicates that the trauma to the head was violent enough to break a bone and perhaps at the same time cause damage to the brain.

A linear skull fracture is the most common type of bony injury [12], occurring with equal frequency in all bones of the skull. Special care should be taken to determine if the fracture line has crossed the area of the middle meningeal artery or the large venous sinuses as hemorrhage may be increased in these cases. The dura may be torn with some linear fractures if there has been separation of the fracture at the time of the injury. Also, leptomeningeal herniation can result with this type of injury. All children with these fractures should be admitted to the local hospital for close observation.

Basal skull fractures are usually not seen on x-ray. The diagnosis, therefore, is usually a clinical conclusion based on suggestive signs such as a cerebrospinal fluid (CSF) leakage from the nose or ears, hemotympanum, mastoid skin bruising (Battle's sign), "raccoon eyes," or scleral hemorrhage. Cranial nerve problems such as hearing loss are also seen.

The vast majority of CSF leaks will resolve spontaneously. When a CSF fistula is present, one must keep watchful for the development of meningitis. The question of administration of antibiotics as a prophylactic measure in these cases is still controversial. No other specific treatment is required, either at the scene of the athletic contest or when the hospital is entered for tertiary care.

All compound or depressed skull fractures require debridement exactly as with any other compound fracture. Antibiotics are usually employed. From a first aid standpoint, these wounds should be covered adequately with a saline- or antibiotic-soaked gauze and the patient expedited to the nearest hospital.

If bone fragments are depressed more than 0.5 cm, they should be elevated. Depressed fractures may often be associated with severe bleeding from the underlying torn venous sinuses. These injuries require referral to a neurosurgeon.

CONCUSSION

This is defined as a temporary alteration of consciousness following trauma to the brain and is usually the result of blunt trauma. Retrograde amnesia is common with this type of injury. The severity of the brain injury correlates roughly with the duration of loss of consciousness or the period of retrograde amnesia.

Normally, no treatment other than observation is needed for concussion and no permanent neurological damage results. There is probably no need to remove athletes from competition for more than

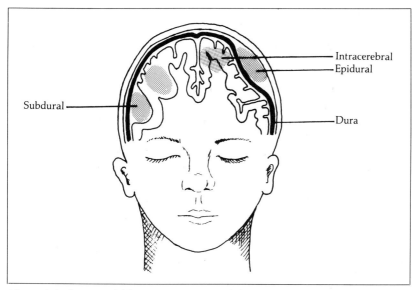

Figure 2-1. Intracranial hematoma may result from any head trauma. Epidural hematoma may lead to rapid neurological deterioration, while subdural or intracranial bleeds may be less dramatic in onset, but equally serious in outcome.

72 hours following concussion unless there are some residual symptoms or he has been concussed repeatedly.

INTRACRANIAL HEMATOMA

This is the most serious consequence of a blunt head injury [12]. Epidural hemorrhage must be diagnosed and treated rapidly if a fatal outcome is to be avoided (Figure 2-1). Pupillary dilatation, hemiparesis, and signs of increased intracranial pressure are the significant characteristics of an intracranial hematoma. Most patients with extradural hemorrhages arrive at surgery within 24 hours of their injury, although in children the signs of extradural hematoma tend to develop more slowly. Surgical decompression is mandatory to relieve the pressure on the brain caused by the hematoma.

Epidural Hematomas

These hematomas occur in the temporal region from a tear of the middle meningeal artery, although 25 percent occur elsewhere. The initial injury is frequently mild and patients often have a normal level of consciousness when first examined although they may have been unconscious initially following the injury. Eighty percent of patients will have a radiologically visible skull fracture. Patients with an expanding hematoma will almost always develop a decrease in their level of consciousness, however, soon after the initial "lucid interval"

[12]. Although this is the classic presentation, many patients with extradural hematomas present in association with more severe injuries may never regain consciousness.

Acute Subdural and Intradural Hematomas

These hematomas are commonly associated with severe head injury and there is usually a continuous alteration in the patient's level of consciousness. Bleeding is venous and is often seen with a contused and lacerated brain. Other manifestations of subdural hematoma may be similar to those of extradural hematoma. Clinical diagnosis is confirmed with CAT scanning or arteriography. Neurosurgical intervention is required and often a craniotomy is necessary to control bleeding and decompress the brain. Because of the underlying brain damage, many survivors are left with permanent disability. Subdural hematomas constitute an important cause of injury in football. Relative brain movements within the helmet during impact result in tears of the subdural connecting veins with resultant hematoma formation.

NECK INJURIES

CERVICAL SPINE INJURIES

Fortunately, cervical spine injuries [25] are relatively uncommon in the athletics of children. Most injuries to the neck region are of the soft tissue variety, usually musculotendinous in nature. These resolve very quickly with only symptomatic treatment. Those cervical spine injuries that occur are often associated with concomitant head injuries—any force violent enough to cause head injury is usually of sufficient magnitude to do damage to the cervical spine. Such injuries, of course, usually follow significant trauma that may occur in high-speed sports such as ice hockey, contact football, or skiing. There are some sports that intrinsically place the cervical spine at definite risk and these include diving, gymnastics, and once again, contact football.

By far, most spinal injuries seen in childhood athletes occur in the cervical area. The most common type of injury is the flexion type where the head and chin are forced downward and forward toward the upper chest. With subsequent posterior ligament rupture and facet joint dislocation, the spinal cord may be injured. At times, a protrusion of the intervertebral disc can occur with little or no bony injury, once again jeopardizing the spinal cord. Hyperextension injuries are less common but may also result in cord injury following dislocation. Direct blows to the top of the skull, which have been seen with diving into shallow water, can cause burst fractures of the vertebra without any dislocation. These injuries result from direct vertical compression forces.

The most important factor in the early recognition of cervical spine injuries is suspicion. If the history is suggestive and the patient complains of pain in the appropriate area, the diagnosis of cervical spine injury should be assumed until proven by roentgenographic examination. All unconscious patients should be treated as if they incurred a cervical spine injury until appropriate x-ray films are obtained. It is necessary to visualize the entire cervical spine. Traction on both arms is usually needed to pull the shoulders caudally in order to visualize the C_7, T_1 junction.

In summary, one must consider the possibility of cervical cord injury with appropriate trauma and great care must be taken in the subsequent handling and transport of patients until a diagnosis is confirmed or proven incorrect [1].

Children are less likely to sustain fractures or dislocation of the cervical spine than adults because their spinal column is much more flexible, but such injuries do occur and the practitioner must be alert so that they will not be missed.

ATLANTAL AXIAL ROTATORY SUBLUXATION

Fifty percent of the rotation of the cervical spine occurs at C_{1-2}. With some twisting injuries, C_{1-2} facet joint becomes locked as the joint is forced to rotate beyond normal range. The child presents with an acute torticollis. This is common in young children, particularly if the child has had a recent sore throat, where adjacent inflammation may have softened the capsule and ligaments of the upper cervical spine. Treatment is usually quite simple with reduction being obtained through continuous Holter traction for approximately 48 hours.

FRACTURES

Compression and burst fractures can occur with direct vertical load; however, they are usually not associated with permanent nerve damage.

Perhaps the most difficult fracture to diagnose adequately is the odontoid fracture. In the younger child, the presence of the epiphyseal plate can be confusing and mistaken for an injury. A quality view through the open mouth and a lateral projection are necessary to view these fractures. Odontoid fractures are treated in traction followed by plaster cast immobilization or a halo-type support.

SUBLUXATION

Forward subluxations of C_2 on C_3 may be seen subsequent to dives or direct blows in collision sports. Reduction is usually obtained by traction with skull tongs, although a halo may also be used for reduction and subsequently incorporated into a cast as a therapeutic measure.

Subluxations or even dislocations can occur virtually in any level of the spine. Due to the increased mobility of the child's cervical spine, however, there may be an appearance of subluxation when actually

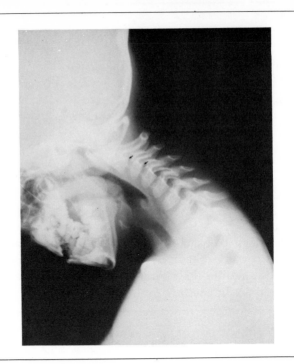

A

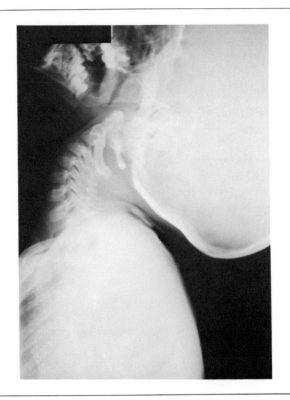

B

the spine is normal. The most frequent area for this false positive diagnosis is at the C_{2-3} level (Figure 2-2).

First and foremost, in the management of these injuries, an adequate history and physical examination must be obtained. One should note carefully if a neurological deficit has occurred. It is important to differentiate between a complete and partial cord injury. Thus, sacral sparing should always be documented. A full x-ray examination with anteroposterior (AP), lateral, and oblique projections should be obtained immediately on entry to a definitive hospital. If these x-rays are normal, then flexion-extension views should be obtained with great caution.

Of vital importance is the initial transfer of the patient from the athletic arena or field. All movements of the neck should be avoided. The neck should be in a neutral position with slight traction maintained until the transfer is complete. The actual, definitive treatment, of course, depends on the injury; indeed, minor injuries can be treated symptomatically or with a soft collar for support. More severe injuries require traction with tongs or halo initially, followed by definitive casting or vesting. Laminectomy is rarely indicated, usually only if there is definite deterioration in neurological function.

It is important to remember that injury to the spinal cord can occur without associated bony injury. Thus, careful initial evaluation is vital and the quality of emergency management will help to avoid major disasters.

INJURIES TO THE RESPIRATORY SYSTEM

The upper airway, thorax, and underlying viscera are areas very prone to athletic injuries [2, 8, 11]. The throat in the child or adolescent is usually prominent and vulnerable, without protection of the large support muscles of the adult. The thoracic cage, very thin and flexible, is likely to allow the force from a concussion or direct blow to be transmitted to the underlying heart or lungs without associated fracture of the ribs or sternum. Some recent equipment modifications, particularly in ice hockey masks, have provided additional throat protection, but they have minimally modified the hazards. Blunt injuries to the larynx, chest wall, and lungs remain common and potentially dangerous in the childhood athlete.

THROAT TRAUMA

Direct trauma to the throat area in young athletes may crack or completely fracture the upper laryngeal and tracheal structures, leaving

---

Figure 2-2. *Lateral flexion (A) and extension (B) views of a 7-year-old child demonstrate the "physiologic" laxity that may be seen at the C_{2-3} or C_{3-4} spinal level in the child, showing no evidence of ligamentous injury.*

the athlete in acute respiratory distress. If, indeed, the airway is displaced, then immediate airway occlusion with cyanosis and subcutaneous emphysema may occur. Although a rare injury, immediate manual reduction of the fracture will restore the airway architecture adequately to allow transfer of the athlete to hospital. Of course, the most common type of upper airway occlusion is from foreign material such as chewing gum. It may also be that the tongue has lodged in the posterior aspect of the throat, perhaps as part of a convulsive episode. The upper airway must be instantly cleared, rendering it patent and functional. If foreign material can be seen, then it can be extracted with a finger or hemostat to provide complete clearance. However, a thrusting adult finger has no place in this particular maneuver; it is likely that the distraught adult, attempting to extract a foreign object from the throat of a child, may awkwardly push the object deeper, making the emergency situation more complicated. Commonly, a firm Heimlich maneuver may forcibly dislodge foreign material from the upper airway. This technique is very rapid and should be well practiced by all medical and paramedical sport personnel. Succinctly, clearing the upper airway is the essential first part of resuscitation.

Rarely, upper airway obstruction may not be relieved by these simple measures and surgical airway entry may be necessary [8, 11]. It is wise to avoid tracheotomy maneuvers on an emergency basis if at all possible. It has been our experience that middle airway entry can be best gained with large-bore sterile needles inserted centrally through the cartilaginous lower tracheal rings. It should be pointed out that this is clearly a rare circumstance and surgical intervention should be reserved as a lifesaving maneuver. Blunt or clumsy instruments, such as pen knives, are to be uniformly condemned.

CHEST TRAUMA

Blunt trauma to the chest wall in the childhood athlete may constitute either a minor contusion or a major visceral rupture [2, 8, 10]. Although minor, a simple chest wall contusion may leave the athlete breathless, frightened, and in considerable pain. Invariably, physical examination reveals normal air entry, but with an increased respiratory rate. This nonemergency situation can be settled with a composed approach to the injured athlete, emphasizing controlled regular breathing. Rolling the young athlete to his side or in a semiprone position greatly facilitates "catching one's breath." If, however, the concussive blow to the chest wall is very severe, it can be followed with considerable worrisome sequelae.

Although it is rather unusual for ribs to be fractured in the adolescent athlete, the situation can occur where multiple ribs do fracture and a flail chest results [10]. These injuries usually are a result of high-velocity trauma in contact sports. Cycling, and occasionally gymnastics, may cause chest wall injury of significant severity. When confronted with an injured gymnast, with either a closed, flail chest or a penetrating rib fracture, the treatment program [10, 11] should be directed to restore the integrity of the functioning rib unit and to control potential hemorrhage within the underlying viscera.

Stabilization of the rib fractures can be accomplished with simple manual pressure, a secured weight, or a circumferential elastic-type wrap. The thoracic wall injury may initially appear to be stable; however, this is usually a manifestation of spasm in the supporting musculature. Clearly, the athlete with this type of injury should be transported to the nearest hospital as quickly as possible after first aid treatment has been administered. Severe chest flailing commonly requires early tracheotomy and positive pressure respiration until the cartilaginous fractures stabilize.

PNEUMOTHORAX

Many children or adolescent athletes participating in many sports possess underlying asymptomatic anomalies of pulmonary parenchyma. Direct blunt chest trauma or excessive exertion can result in a pneumothorax (Figure 2-3). The pneumothorax may range in severity from a very mild air leak manifested with minor respiratory stress or a massive pneumothorax, resulting in a startling clinical picture of respiratory distress, cyanosis, and even altered consciousness. If the pneumothorax is allowed to progress unattended while the athlete is awaiting transfer to a hospital, he or she may not survive. The immediate insertion of a chest tube is mandatory. This tube may be the traditional chest tube or it may be substituted for by multiple large-bore needles inserted in the second rib interspace along the midclavicular line. If the tracheal shift does not immediately indicate the lung that is malfunctioning, then both thoracic cavities should be penetrated.

HEMOTHORAX

Hemothorax is rather unusual as a result of athletic trauma and is usually secondary to a laceration of the lung or frank bleeding from the chest wail [11, 20]. If the hemothorax is severe, then the young athlete will demonstrate early shock and hampered respiration. If this injury is suspected, immediate hospital attention is necessary.

INJURY TO THE DIAPHRAGM

Ruptures of the diaphragm usually follow severe motor vehicle trauma; however, some literature reviews have reported 25 percent occurring as a result of athletics [1a, 29]. These injuries are usually caused by a direct concussion to the lower ribs or abdomen that forces a rent in the left hemidiaphragm. These youngsters may demonstrate imme-

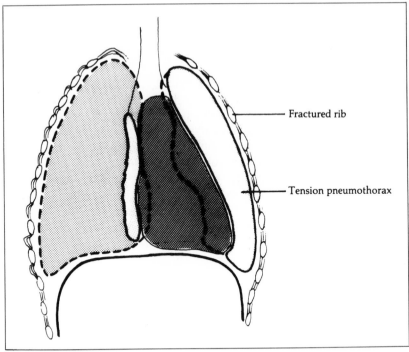

Figure 2-3. A tension pneumothorax may result from blunt trauma to the chest with fractured ribs.

diate cardiopulmonary distress as major viscera enter the chest cavity and impair normal cardiac and lung filling. Most frequently, however the young athlete presents with moderate left chest wall pain from the direct blow combined with very little, if any, breathing difficulties. However, over the next few days or weeks, the young athlete develops gastrointestinal, respiratory, or even cardiac impairment. At this point, clinical and radiological examination will illuminate the diagnosis. The most devastating injury, which produces a severe diaphragmatic rupture with migration of the abdominal viscera to the thorax, normally requires emergency attention to restore pulmonary function. Specifically, mouth-to-mouth positive pressure ventilation may be necessary. Vomiting is extremely common following this type of insult and should be treated with positioning and a plastic airway if it is available. The earliest possible transfer to the tertiary care hospital is necessary for definitive surgical management.

CARDIAC INJURIES
Life-threatening sport injuries related to the heart are rare; however, recent medical and media reports have cited instances of cardiac in-

juries in young athletes that have been associated with a profound delay in diagnosis and definitive management [2, 13, 15, 17, 24, 28]. Indeed, the most common reason for this tardy treatment invariably has been the lack of suspicion about cardiac injury on the part of the treating medical team.

PENETRATION OF THE MYOCARDIUM

Obviously, the penetrating cardiac wound poses less of a diagnostic challenge than the blunt injury. In athletics, these type of open injuries are most uncommon and usually are bizarre in etiology. They usually occur in high-velocity sports that include the use of poles or sticks. Skiers are particularly vulnerable, and it seems that a falling horseback rider is also at relatively high risk. The clinical picture usually reveals profound shock and many of those injured die before reaching the emergency room at a hospital. If confronted with such an athlete, obviously having been impaled on a sharp object, it is inadvisable to remove the device until tertiary resuscitative measures are available. If there has been a rent in the myocardium, then to remove the penetrating implement invites disaster.

MYOCARDIAL CONTUSION

Direct blows to the chest wall are extremely frequent in all sports. The growing athlete, whether playing a contact or a noncontact recreational sport, is at significant risk. In our geographical area, soccer, ice hockey, and even basketball are the sports most frequently responsible for blunt trauma to the chest.

It is mandatory that the sport medicine physician and paramedical sport personnel develop a high level of suspicion when treating the apparently benign chest bruise.

The growing athlete is particularly vulnerable and prone to contusion of the myocardium. The rib cage, as previously mentioned, and supporting chest wall musculatures constitute architecturally a very elastic shield for the heart and lung. Indeed, the cardiac literature has suggested that fractured ribs can be a good prognostic sign in the growing athlete because they suggest that much of the force has been dissipated before it reaches the chest organs [17]. The adolescent athlete absorbs the blow through an elastic rib cage that rarely fractures and, thus, usually transmits the force of the blow to the heart and lungs.

Once the myocardium has accepted this exogenous force, a variety of conditions may follow. A pericardial effusion may result and cardiac tamponade may slowly or rapidly occur The pericardial sac in the child is very small and will accept much less than the 200 ml necessary to produce cardiac tamponade in the adult [17].

To complicate matters even further, it is sometimes most difficult to clinically evaluate the young athlete with accuracy using adult diagnostic equipment. A large blood pressure cuff, for instance, may be a major hindrance in an attempt to ascertain the vital signs on a thrashing youngster who is in obvious pain. Vital signs can be very labile in children and the childhood athlete generally tends to have a lower blood pressure than the adult. These variables complicate further the clinical assessment [17, 24].

CARDIAC TAMPONADE

Cardiac tamponade secondary to myocardial contusion is difficult to diagnose and is rarely suspected, but it is a life-threatening situation if not treated expeditiously. Heart sounds are usually muffled, and are difficult to evaluate, particularly with the extraneous noise of an athletic crowd. The venous pressure elevation is virtually impossible to evaluate in an emotionally distraught, adolescent athlete. Thus, with these difficulties, it is vital to suspect tamponade whenever shock is unaccompanied by evidence of obvious outward bleeding. This situation is clearly a surgical emergency and rapid transport to a hospital is essential. At the scene, however, lifesaving pericardiocentesis may be necessary, and can be performed with a large-bore needle through a xiphisternal stab. Even within the hospital setting, diagnosis may be difficult, as the classical distortion of the cardiac silhouette may not always be present in children. Serial electrocardiograms and enzyme changes likewise have been found to be inconsistent. Definitive and successful management is achieved when the evaluations of these multiple clinical and laboratory variables are merged.

CARDIAC ARRHYTHMIA

Cardiac arrhythmia may occur in child and adolescent athletes for a variety of reasons. Indeed, cardiac contusion is usually the most common triggering injury, but the youngster may also have an endogenous feature of predisposition, such as a congenital heart defect or an aberration of the electrical conducting system. When a youngster develops a cardiac arrhythmia during an athletic contest, it is most fortunate if the attending personnel are skilled in cardiopulmonary resuscitation. At a minimum, though, available oxygen, defibrillation equipment, and some pharmaceuticals may be necessary for successful emergency resuscitation. Not uncommonly however, valuable time better spent transporting the injured child to a hospital center may be lost by well-intentioned, but ill-qualified personnel attempting to use unfamiliar equipment and techniques at the scene. Oxygen, administered by an Ambu bag with an appropriate plastic airway, is usually sufficient to maintain respiration while the patient is transferred to hospital. This technique is superior to a difficult and prolonged intubation attempted on a thrashing child.

All sport medical and paramedical personnel should be trained and qualified in cardiopulmonary resuscitation (CPR). The chief medical officer responsible for the athletic contest must organize the support personnel in order that they may execute quality first-aid treatment, emergency management, and ultimate transfer of the injured competitor.

UROLOGICAL INJURIES

Injuries to the urinary tract of any magnitude are uncommon in athletics. Nonetheless, they must be considered if there has been significant abdominal trauma [4, 19, 22]. Kidneys and distended bladders may be ruptured by what seems to be a trivial blow. The kidneys are the internal organs most frequently injured in children, even more commonly damaged than the spleen (Figure 2-4). However, one must bear in mind that injuries to other organs often accompany renal injury. In athletic endeavors, most renal injuries follow blunt trauma— penetrating injuries are exceedingly rare. Approximately 10 percent of children sustaining renal injuries have some preexisting renal abnormality. Injuries to the lower urinary tract are usually secondary to pelvic trauma and, therefore, are not usually seen by those treating athletic injuries. Ureteral injuries are secondary to either penetrating

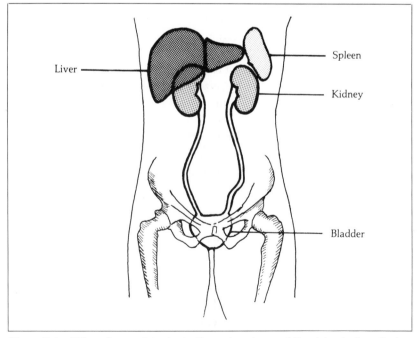

Figure 2-4. Although rare, injuries to the major viscera of the abdominal cavity in the child can be life-threatening.

wounds or blunt trauma and are often associated with fractures of the transverse process of a lumbar vertebra. Bladder injuries occur with concomitant pelvic fractures [9]. A full, distended bladder can rupture with blunt trauma, spilling urine directly into the peritoneal cavity, resulting in peritoneal irritation. Extravasation of the urine can also be extraperitoneal; in this instance, clinical signs may be less obvious and roentgenographic investigation will be required for diagnosis. Urethral injuries following accidents are nearly always seen in association with pelvic fractures.

Renal injuries are usually associated with flank tenderness, with or without a palpable mass. The cardinal sign of any urinary tract injury is hematuria. However, the amount of blood in the urine does not necessarily correlate with the severity of the injury. Many minor injuries have gross hematuria and more significant injuries produce only a few red cells in the urine.

Renal Injuries

Simple contusions are the most common renal injuries. The kidney parenchyma is bruised, but no other injury occurs; thus, treatment is purely symptomatic. Contusions may be associated with rupture of the surrounding capsule resulting in blood escaping into the perirenal area forming a hematoma. These injuries will also resolve without surgical intervention, leaving no residual effects.

If the collecting system is damaged, extravasation of urine will be seen on the intravenous pyelogram. These patients will require surgical intervention to repair the defect to provide adequate drainage. Failure to make the diagnosis of extravasation of urine will probably result in an unsalvageable kidney, due to intense scarring or abscess formation. Surgery is not usually performed on an emergency basis, but rather a few days later when bleeding is more easily controlled and the necrotic tissue more easily recognized.

Vascular injuries are most uncommon in nonpenetrating injuries. But if they occur, they present true surgical emergencies, necessitating immediate operation in order to salvage the affected kidney. The intravenous pyelogram (IVP) examination will demonstrate a lack of contrast material with these types of injuries.

Ureteral, Bladder, and Urethral Injuries

The important thing to bear in mind with these injuries [4] is that at times they are exceedingly difficult to diagnose and must be suspected in the injured athlete. Surgical treatment of these lesions involves advanced urological techniques [22, 27]. When definitive treatment is available, intravenous pyelograms are invaluable as part of the initial evaluation of the young athlete suspected of having a urinary tract injury. With urethral injuries in the male, heralded by blood in the meatus, catheterization should not be performed. A urethrogram is indicated in the emergency room, followed by suprapubic drainage if the urethrogram is positive.

INJURIES TO EXTERNAL MALE GENITALIA

Although there are a multitude of conditions that affect the male genitalia, the injuries of concern to the sports medicine practitioner are those resulting from direct blows. Small hematomas should be treated with rest, support, and application of ice until resolution is complete. More severe trauma may cause testicular rupture with subsequent hematocele formation requiring surgical exploration.

The key to successful treatment of urological injuries is, of course, an accurate and precise diagnosis. The appropriate use of intravenous pyelography, cystography, and urethrography cannot be over emphasized.

Urinary catheters are contraindicated in all cases of suspected urinary tract damage, except with urethral tears, when a suprapubic cystostomy should be performed. This enables one to monitor urinary output and to evaluate the urine for bleeding.

The indications for surgery are few. They include extravasation of the urine, vascular damage as seen by arteriography, and the presence of massive hemorrhage uncontrollable by nonoperative means.

ABDOMINAL INJURIES

Young athletes frequently absorb blunt trauma to the lower thorax and abdominal areas. Most commonly, contact sports are the major culprits. This is not to say, though, that even less "dangerous" sports, such as baseball, cannot be a triggering source. Very rarely, however, does a blow to the abdomen result in significant injury to the underlying viscera necessitating emergency medical attention. But such an injury requires prompt action.

The stomach, duodenum, and even lower bowel may be perforated as a consequence of a high-velocity blow or fall [7, 18]. Penetrating injuries, of course, are exceedingly remote in children in sports and usually result from a fall on a sharp object or playing implement. Indeed a ruptured viscus may be a major diagnostic problem as in, for instance, the case of a ruptured duodenum. This structure exists virtually totally retroperitoneally, thus clinical guarding and peritonism can be very late signs. Injuries to the spleen will be the source of most abdominal emergencies in children's sports [5, 14, 16, 21]. The rib cage in the child, as previously noted, is extremely flexible and can transmit a major force to the spleen. With rupture, a catastrophic picture may occur with hypovolemic shock. The child may complain of dizziness and lightheadedness, progressing abruptly to complete vascular collapse. It is vital to be aware of the young athlete who has taken a rather sharp elbow to the rib cage during basketball and complains of shoulder pain. Very commonly, this radiating pain heralds hemorrhage from the spleen (see Figure 2-4).

Simply, any youngster participating in sports who has incurred a direct blow to the abdomen must be observed very carefully. If pain persists after the contest, then medical observation in a hospital setting is indicated. During a game, any athlete who continues to complain of abdominal pain after injury must not be allowed to continue until the clinical problem resolves.

MUSCULOSKELETAL AND PERIPHERAL VASCULAR INJURIES

Fractures are commonplace, usually readily diagnosed, and in most instances, are treated expertly by the family physician [3, 6, 26]. However, even the most innocent-appearing fracture presents potential hazards that are feared by the most expert traumatologist.

Assume that an 8-year-old ice hockey player is jammed against the goalpost and incurs a forced valgus stress to his knee. The youngster appreciates instant pain to the knee and falls to the ice. Physical examination by the attending doctor reveals a knee angled at approximately 45 degrees with normal vascular status and absence of compounding or skin breakdown. Since it is realized, statistically, that in the growing skeleton, the supporting ligaments are stronger than the growth plate, the leg deformity is probably secondary to a fracture of the epiphyseal plate.

When faced with such circumstance, the physician or paramedical person at the game must consider these vital elements: (1) What first aid measures should be administered? (2) Can manipulation of the fracture be done safely to facilitate transfer to the hospital for definitive management?

Indeed, when one is confronted with an athlete who obviously has suffered a fractured extremity that is deformed, then the leg or arm should be splinted as it lies and the patient transported as rapidly as possible to a tertiary care unit. This rule assumes that the pulses in the extremity are normal. If, however, the fractured and deformed arm or leg is pulseless, then clearly, the limb must be gently manipulated in order to restore alignment before transfer.

When reducing such a fracture of the arm or leg, the extremity is gently cradled and gradual, progressive traction is applied with manual counter-traction. At no time should force be applied abruptly, with traction being offered progressively, gently and consistently. The limb should be restored to its anatomical position or as close as possible to anatomical position. Unnecessary time should not be wasted in waiting for sedatives or appliances. This technique of manipulation should be abandoned after a ten-minute period. That is to suggest that unnecessary time on repeated reduction should not be wasted at the time of the athletic injury.

Compound fractures are always a concern and should be considered emergencies. Any time direct contact is made between the bone and the exterior, sterile dressings should be applied over the wound and the athlete transferred to hospital. If wound compounding occurs simultaneously with a deformed pulseless limb, then clearly, the leg must be reduced into a more normal attitude of anatomy as restoration of blood supply is the priority.

Fractures with vascular injuries are certainly rare, but even a single episode ill-treated can lead to devastating sequelae.

Sports injuries are second only to high-speed motor vehicle trauma as the cause of skeletal injury with associated vascular trauma. High-risk sports include football, soccer, cycling, and skiing. High-velocity impact is usually necessary to produce a vascular insult and, commonly, the injury to the vessel has exposed the artery to a tension stress.

Regarding the issue of vascular injury, one should remain constantly concerned with the vessel compression that can occur secondary to pressure outside of the lumen [23]. For example, young athletes with a supracondylar fracture of the humerus are at considerable risk in developing arterial and venous obstruction secondary to an expanding hematoma. If the pressure is allowed to reach a critical level above arterial pressure, the forearm intracompartmental pressure will increase and result in muscle ischemia. This type of compartment syndrome may occur in the arm or the leg and must be treated with expedition and thorough compartment decompression. Such decompression may be accomplished with ice and elevation, but in many instances, formal fasciotomies are necessary. Be aware of the child who suffers with inordinate pain after a fracture or a significant soft tissue injury to the upper or lower extremity. Be aware also of the child who was treated with a circumferential bandage or cast for a fracture or contusion of the extremity. More specifically, the physical findings may be most misleading because a complete deep compartment infarction may occur in the face of normal pulses. The most consistent clinical features of an impending compartment syndrome include inordinate pain, sensory dysesthesia, and pain with passive extension of fingers and plantar flexion of the foot depending on the compartment.

With any type of injury to the arm or leg, be it skeletal or soft tissue, it is mandatory to employ half-splints and padding rather than circumferential casts or bandages. After the injury is treated, even at the game site, the athlete should be encouraged to see his family doctor the next morning. If the pain becomes too severe and uncontrolled with aspirin, therapy, and elevation, hospital attention is required immediately.

REFERENCES

1. American Academy of Orthopaedic Surgeons. *Emergency Care and Transportation of the Sick and Injured.* Chicago: American Academy of Orthopaedic Surgeons, 1971.
1a. Andrus, C. H., and Morton, J. H.   Rupture of the diaphragm after blunt trauma. *Am. J. Surg.*119:686, 1970.
2. Blair, E., et al.   Major blunt chest trauma. *Curr. Probl. Surg.* 2:64, 1969.
3. Boyd, D. R.   Trauma, a controllable disease in the 1980s. *J. Trauma* 20:14, 1979.
4. Burns, E.   Injuries of the lower urinary tract. *J.A.M.A.* 184:688, 1963.
5. Burrington, J. D.   Surgical repair of a ruptured spleen in children. *Arch. Surg.* 112:417, 1977.
6. Cave, E. F., Burke, J. F. and Boyd, R. J.   *Trauma Management.* Chicago: Year Book, 1974.
7. Cleveland, H. C., and Wadell, W. R.   Retroperitoneal rupture of the duodenum due to non-penetrating trauma. *Surg. Clin. North Am.* 43:413, 1963.
8. Cohn, R.   Non-penetrating wounds of the lungs and bronchi. *Surg. Clin. North Am.* 52:585, 1972.
9. Conolly, W. B.   Observations on fractures of the pelvis. *J. Trauma* 9:104, 1969.
10. Cullen, P., et al.   Treatment of flail chest. *Arch. Surg.* 110:1099, 1975.
11. Craighead, C. C., and Glass, B. A.   Management of non-penetrating injuries of the chest. *J.A.M.A.* 104:1138, 1960.
12. Davis, L. E.   Trauma, Management of Acutely Injured Patient and Section 41—Neurosurgery. In D. Sabiston, Jr. (Ed.), *Textbook of Surgery* (10th ed.). Philadelphia: Saunders, 1972.
13. DeMuth, W. E., Jr., and Zinsser, H. F., Jr.   Myocardial contusion. *Arch. Intern. Med.* 115:434, 1965.
14. Douglas, G. A., and Simpson, J. S.   The conservative management of splenic trauma. *J. Pediatr. Surg.* 6:565, 1971.
15. Drapanas, T., and Jones, J. C.   Cardiac contusion, a capricious syndrome. *Ann. Surg.* 181:567, 1975.
16. Erickson, W. D., Burgert, E. O., and Lynn, H. B.   Hazard of infection following splenectomy in children. *Am. J. Dis. Child.* 116:1, 1968.
17. Golladay, E. S.   Special problems of cardiac injuries in infants and children. *J. Trauma* 19:526, 1979.
18. Harrison, R. C., and Debas, H. T.   Injuries of stomach and duodenum. *Surg. Clin. North Am.* 52:635, 1972.
19. Kaufman, J. J., and Brosman, S. A.   Blunt injuries of the genitourinary tract. *Surg. Clin. North Am.* 52:747, 1972.
20. Maloney, J. V.   The conservative management of traumatic haemothorax. *Am. J. Surg.* 93:523, 1957.
21. Mishalany, H.   Repair of the ruptured spleen. *J. Pediatr. Surg.* 9:175, 1974.
22. Morrow, J. W., and Mendez, R.   Renal trauma. *J. Urol.* 104:649, 1970.
23. Murbarak, S. J., and Carroll, N. C.   Volkmann's contracture in children: aetiology and prevention. *J. Bone Joint Surg. [Br.]* 61:285, 1979.
24. Roe, B. B.   Cardiac trauma including injury of great vessels. *Surg. Clin. North Am.* 52:573, 1972.
25. Rothman, R. H., and Simeone, F. A. *The Spine.* Philadelphia:Saunders, 1975.

26. Sharrard, W. J. W. *Pediatric Orthopaedics and Fractures.* Oxford, England: Blackwell, 1971.
27. Touloukian, R. J. *Pediatric Surgery.* Chicago: Year Book, 1979.
28. Trinkle, J. K., et al. Management of the wounded heart. *Ann. Thorac. Surg.* 17:233, 1974.
29. Wren, H. B., et al. Traumatic rupture of the diaphragm. *J. Trauma* 2:117, 1962.

3. Preparticipation Evaluation and First Aid for Sports

Lyle J. Micheli and John G. Yost

The physician's role in the care of young athletes entails a three-fold obligation: prevention of injuries, diagnosis and treatment of injuries, and rehabilitation of injuries [6].

The preparticipation medical evaluation is the cornerstone of the physician's care of young athletes [1]. The preparticipation evaluation of children or adolescents interested in sports participation provides an excellent opportunity not only to assess their physical capabilities but also to perform a good overall health assessment. This assessment can include screening for incipient diseases such as hypertension, diabetes, allergies; detection of possible physical handicaps; and careful reexamination of sites of previous injury [5]. The exact organization of the preparticipation evaluation is a matter of some debate. Opinions vary as to whether this is best done by the family physician or the team physician [1, 3, 6, 9]. If there is no specific team physician, of course, the pediatrician or family physician must be prepared to accept responsibility for this evaluation. If there is a designated team physician, it is indeed useful for him or her to participate in the preparticipation evaluation, both as a means of getting to know the athletes and sports staff and of becoming aware of any particular problems the young athletes may have.

The goals of the preparticipation evaluation in children include assessing the overall health of the child, including detecting conditions that might eliminate the child from competition; anthropometric measurements, including height, weight, and percentage of body weight as fat; determining the child's specific fitness for the sport in question, and determining the child's relative level of maturation, as a help in sports counseling [2, 6].

In our experience, the ideal setting for the preparticipation evaluation is a health facility or clinic, where it is possible to set up a number of different stations [6]. We have usually set up four different types of stations. The first is used to obtain basic vital signs, height, weight, and skin caliper measurements for assessment of body fat, as well as an initial review of the medical history. This is usually quite adequately staffed by school nurses or athletic trainers. The second station is used to perform a general medical examination and it is usually manned by pediatricians or general physicians. The third station is for the specific assessment of the musculoskeletal system including the spine, torso, and extremities and is usually manned by orthopedic surgeons. The final station is for specific assessment of athletic fitness and includes functional tests such as a standing jump, step testing, or even treadmill testing or distance running, pull-ups, or push-ups, and sit-ups. Finally, the overall results of the assessment are discussed with the student with particular attention to conditions that must be corrected or rehabilitated before participation will be allowed.

Opinion as to when the comprehensive preparticipation evaluation should be done varies [1, 6, 9]. We feel the examination should be done 3 to 4 months prior to the beginning of the fall season. This leaves time to evaluate and correct specific problems and can allow the athlete to participate sooner. To have examinations prior to each season is both time-consuming and costly, with little yield. Accumulative records of injuries, illnesses, and medical care would be sufficient to identify those who are in need of medical attention before a different sport is undertaken. The emphasis should be on quality not on frequency [9]. The following equipment is needed [10]:

1. Assembly area (gym or locker room) with numbered stations
2. Examination room (coach's office)
3. Table (two: one for cardiovascular/abdominal, one for orthopedic)
4. Examination forms
5. Pencils (red and black)
6. Snellen chart
7. Tongue depressors
8. Flashlight
9. Oto-ophthalmoscope
10. Stethoscope
11. Paper cups
12. "Lab-Stix"
13. Blood pressure cuff
14. Reflex hammer
15. Tape measure
16. Pin
17. "Fat-o-meter"

THE MEDICAL HISTORY

The screening medical history is perhaps the single most important portion of the health appraisal [9]. The screening history should draw attention to illnesses, injuries, and operations that have a significant bearing on potential ability or are contraindications to vigorous activity. This will also help to bring to the physician's attention any past injuries not previously noted—the example most frequently given is of a fracture of the carponavicular bone that escaped initial diagnosis. The screening history will aid the physician in determining present control of medical problems and whether the athlete is knowledgeable about

MEDICAL EVALUATION FOR SPORTS

HISTORY

1. Name _____

2. Social security number _____

3. Home address _____
              Number and Street   City   State   Zip

4. Phone _____ 5. Sex _____ 6. Age _____

7. Date of birth _____ 8. Marital status _____

9. Present team _____

10. Level of competition: (a) professional (b) college (c) high school
    (d) varsity (e) junior varsity

11. Whom shall we notify in case of an emergency? Name _____
    Relation _____ Address _____
    Phone _____ Business phone _____

12. Health insurance: Name _____
    Names of persons insured _____
    Policy number _____

13. During participation, do you wear (a) contact lenses (b) glasses
    (c) dental appliances (d) mouth protector

DISEASES AND ILLNESSES (PAST AND PRESENT) Circle number of all appropriate conditions	Details of circled conditions
14. 1 Congenital generalized abnormalities or absent organs	
2 Blood disease	
3 Infectious mononucleosis, pneumonia, or others	
4 Epilepsy	
5 Hepatitis, jaundice	
6 Diabetes	
7 Sugar, albumin, pus, blood in urine	
8 Cough up blood	
9 Allergies (to drugs, etc.)	
10 High blood pressure	
11 Concussion or knocked out (give number)	
12 Recurring headaches or blackouts	
13 Blurred vision, sties, pink eye	
14 Chronic nose bleeds	
15 Skin infections, boils, impetigo, etc.	

Figure 3-1. Representative medical history for sports competition. (Reprinted by permission from the New York State Journal of Medicine, *copyright by the Medical Society of New York. From J. L. Marshall and H. M. Tischler, Screening for sports, guidelines.* New York J. Med. 78:243, 1978.)

16	Congenital heart disease, rheumatic fever, murmurs
17	Appendicitis, hernia
18	Chest pain during exercise
19	Tuberculosis
20	Chronic cough
21	Frequent indigestion, heartburn
22	Ulcer (location)
23	Kidney or bladder diseases
24	Heat exhaustion or heat stroke
25	Hearing problems
26	Mental illness
27	Any other illness not listed

15. Are you presently taking medication? What kind? _____
What dosage? _____

16. Operations or hospitalizations
Type   Date   Hospital   Doctor's Name and Address

17. Any diagnostic tests performed? EKG, EEG, EMG, arthrogram, etc? _____

18. Bones and joints (orthopaedic history): Circle where applicable
    1. Head   7. Ribs
    2. Neck   8. Hips and pelvis
    3. Shoulder-clavicle   9. Thigh
    4. Arm, elbow, wrist   10. Knee, kneecap
    5. Hand   11. Leg
    6. Spine   12. Ankle
                               13. Foot
    Details of circled regions (explain type of injury or condition, i.e.,
    arthritis, calcium deposits, nerve injury, fracture)

19. Do you have any bone grafts, spinal fusions, plates, screws, etc.?

20. Do you wear any type of brace, splint, or orthopaedic appliance?

_____

FEMALE SUPPLEMENT

21. Menstrual history: Age of onset _____ Interval _____ Duration _____

22. Conditions: (a) dysmenorrhea   (b) varicose veins   (c) birth control pills
    (d) pregnancy   (e) other _____

_____

I hereby state that, to the best of my knowledge and belief, my answers to
the foregoing questions are correct.

_____   _____
Signature   Date

his condition. History can be compiled by the athlete under the guidance of a school nurse prior to the physical exam. The presence of a school nurse with cumulative school medical records will help to ensure an accurate history and serve as a source of information concerning immunizations. The medical history should be reviewed by a physician or nurse so any need for special attention will be identified [3, 6]. An excellent representative history is listed in Figure 3-1.

PHYSICAL EXAMINATION, INCLUDING MUSCULOSKELETAL PROFILE

The physical examination should be simple but complete. It is designed for a screening purpose but should also be used to determine general health and fitness. In performing the examination on candidates for sports it is important to think of them as boys and girls and not simply as potential athletes. The initial examination of a child who is a first-time candidate for sports activities should be more than a screening process—it also should provide an opportunity to detect existing congenitally acquired health problems and to do health counseling [6]. A child athlete offers the most potential for accomplishing something meaningful in the preparticipation examination. As athletes become more experienced, one is less likely to discover significant medical problems during the course of an examination. Later in the athlete's career one usually looks for only the residual of previous injuries. For the experienced athlete, the examination serves primarily as a quality control with treatment and rehabilitation of previous injuries [11]. A more detailed examination of a particular system or extremity can be performed if indicated by the history. Also the screening examination may be the first time a particular problem presents to the physician, e.g., scoliosis, undiagnosed heart murmur, single testicle, or knee instability [3], and appropriate consultation can be recommended.

Height, weight, and age should be noted initially. The Snellen test for visual acuity is recommended. Determination of blood pressure is also done by nurse or trainer with attention drawn to poor vision or a diastolic blood pressure above the 95th percentile for age [10]. Examination of skin and scalp for pustular acne, herpes, or athlete's foot may be done by the physician, nurse or trainer. Examination of the musculoskeletal system will be discussed separately.

Examination of the eyes should check for equal pupils and evidence of old injury. The mouth examination should check for prosthesis and dental caries. The neck, chest, and abdomen should be examined by a physician. Organomegaly, cardiac murmurs, lack of paired organs (including testes) and lymphadenopathy must be noted. An evaluation of percentage of body fat should be obtained. We recommend the "fat-o-meter" for quick accurate measurement of percentage of body fat. Also evaluation of physiologic maturity should be done, utilizing either Tanner's stages of development of maturation, or hand and

GENERAL PHYSICAL EXAMINATION

(To be filled out by physician)
1. Name _____ 2. HT _____ 3. WT _____ 4. BP __/__
5. Pulse _____ Normal reading after 1 minute of running _____
6. Vision: Without glasses: R ___ L ___; With glasses/lenses: R ___ L_____
7. Hearing: R _____/15   L _____/15
8. Skin: (a) dry (b) moist (c) coarse (d) smooth (e) rash (f) scars
          (g) nail changes (h) telangiectasia (i) discoloration (j) needle
          tracks (k) other _____
9. Scalp: (a) normal (b) tenderness (c) scar (d) other _____
10. Lymph nodes: (a) normal (b) absent (c) location _____
11. Ears (pinna, external canal, tympanic membrane): (a) normal (b) discharge
          (c) other _____
12. Nose (septum, sinus): (a) normal (b) tenderness (c) obstruction
          (d) discharge (e) other _____
13. Throat and mouth (lips, tonsils, buccal mucosa, tongue, pharynx, teeth,
          gums): (a) normal   (b) abnormal
14. Neck (thyroid, trachea): (a) normal (b) mass (c) other _____
15. Chest and lungs: Inspection: (a) normal   (b) abnormal
                    Auscultation: (a) normal   (b) abnormal
16. Heart: Auscultation: (a) normal   (b) abnormal
17. Spine: (a) normal (b) lordosis (c) kyphosis (d) scoliosis
18. Abdomen (liver, spleen, kidneys, stomach, appendix, intestines):
          Inspection: (a) flat (b) distended (c) scaphoid (d) scars
          (e) other _____
          Palpation: (a) normal (b) rigid (c) tender (d) mass (e) rebound
          (f) fluid wave (g) hernia
19. Genitalia: (a) normal (b) scrotal mass (c) edema (d) tenderness
          (e) epididymus (f) penile lesion (g) discharge (h) evidence of
          surgery (i) other
20. Nervous system and reflexes: Pupils: (a) equal (b) unequal
          Knee jerk: (a) normal   (b) abnormal
          Ankle jerk: (a) normal   (b) abnormal
          Romberg test: (a) normal   (b) abnormal
21. Immunizations: Flu ____/____/____ Tetanus _____ Polio _____ Rubella ___
22. Lab studies: Albumin _____ Specific gravity _____
          Urine: Glucose _____ Other _____
          Blood: CBC _____ Blood sugar _____ Sickle cell _____
          Other _____
23. Special studies
          (a) Chest and other x-ray findings _____
          _____
          (b) EKG/ECG stress test _____
          (c) EMG _____
          (d) Muscle tests _____
          _____
          (e) Fitness evaluation _____
          _____

*Figure 3-2. Representative general physical examination for sports competition.
(Reprinted by permission from the New York State Journal of Medicine,
copyright by the Medical Society of the State of New York. From J. L. Marshall
and H. M. Tischler, Screening for sports, guidelines. New York J. Med. 78:243,
1978.)*

MUSCULOSKELETAL EXAMINATION

1. Neck: (a) normal (b) pain in range of motion (c) limited rotation
   (d) limited flexion (e) limited extension

2. Spine: (a) normal (b) excess lordosis (c) kyphosis (d) scoliosis (e) limited
   motion (f) pain with motion (g) decreased reflexes (h) sensory
   change (i) increased weakness (j) + Leseque's

3. Shoulder: (a) normal (b) limited range of motion (c) pain throughout
   range of motion (d) pain and limited range of motion
   (e) atrophy

4. Elbow: (a) normal (absence of hyperextension, i.e., extension = 180°)
   (b) hyperextension (>180°) (c) flexion contracture (<180°)

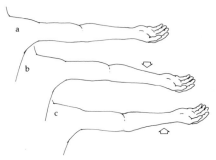

5. Wrist: (a) normal (b) limited range of motion (c) pain with motion

6. M-P extension: (a) <70° (b) 70–89° (c) = 90° (d) >90°

7. Thumb-forearm: (a) >45°
   (b) 1–45°, not touching
   (c) +
   (d) + +
   (e) does not apply

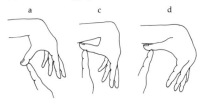

8. Hand: (a) normal (b) limited in flexion (c) limited in extension (d) limited
   in rotation (e) pain in flexion (f) pain in extension (g) pain in
   rotation

9. Functional tests (score: 0 = cannot perform, 1 = can perform with
   discomfort, 2 = can perform well):
   (a) up and down stairs _____(b) running in place _____
   (c) hop on one leg _____ (d) half squat _____ (e) full squat _____

*Figure 3-3. Representative musculoskeletal examination for sports competition.
(Reprinted by permission from the* New York State Journal of Medicine, *copyright by the Medical Society of the State of New York. From J. L. Marshall and H. M. Tischler, Screening for sports, guidelines.* New York J. Med. *78:243, 1978.)*

10. Palms to floor: (a) >10 inches from floor
    (b) <10 inches from floor
    (c) tips to floor
    (d) fingers to floor
    (e) palms to floor

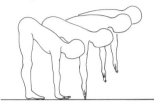

11. Hip: (a) normal (b) limited in flexion (c) limited in extension (d) limited in rotation (e) pain in flexion (f) pain in extension (g) pain in rotation

12. Knee alignment: (a) varus
    (b) valgus, 0–14° normal
    (c) valgus, >15°
    (d) flexion contracture
    (e) normal
    (f) hyperextension

    Range of motion: (a) normal (b) limited in flexion or extension (c) limited in flexion and extension (d) <90°

    Thigh sizes: (a) equal (b)1- to 2-cm difference (c) >2-cm difference

    Stability (for all stability scores, answer must include both number and letter):

(A) LCL (5) Normal = opposite leg
         (4) Mild instability in flexion
         (3) Moderate instability in flexion
         (2) Instability in flexion and extension
         (0) Gross instability
             (a) Hard end point
             (b) Soft end point

(B) MCL (5) Normal = opposite leg
         (4) Mild instability in flexion
         (3) Moderate instability in flexion
         (2) Instability in flexion and extension
         (0) Gross instability
             (a) Hard end point
             (b) Soft end point

(C) ACL (anterior drawer sign)*:
         (5) Normal = opposite leg
         (4) Slight jog
         (3) Moderate jog
         (2) Severe in neutral
         (0) Severe in neutral and rotation
             (a) Hard end point
             (b) Soft end point

(D) PCL (posterior drawer sign)*:
         (5) Normal = opposite leg
         (4) Slight jog
         (3) Moderate jog
         (2) Severe in neutral
         (0) Severe in neutral and rotation
             (a) Hard end point
             (b) Soft end point

*Test to derive score

Palpation
Scar: (a) yes (b) no
Pain: (a) yes (b) no
Effusion: (a) yes (b) no
Soft tissue swelling: (a) yes (b) no
McMurray, Appley, Snap: (a) yes (b) no

13. Patella
Pain: (a) yes (b) no
Excursion: (a) ½ inch (b) 1 inch (c) 1–1½ inches (d) 2 inches (e) >2 inches
Displacement: (a) medial (b) lateral (c) straight
Apprehension test: (a) yes (b) no
Crepitation: (a) yes (b) no

14. Ankle: Range of motion: (a) normal (b) limited (c) painful
Stability: (a) normal (b) + anterior drawer sign
(c) + medial/lateral talar shift
Heel cord tightness: (a) >90° (b) 90° (c) <90°

15. Feet: (a) pes cavus (high arches)
(b) normal
(c) splay
(d) flat (pes planus)
(e) pronated

16. Examiner's impression (diagnosis)

17. Recommendations

18. Examiner _____

Figure 3-3 (continued)

wrist x-rays with a Greulich and Pyle Atlan, or a dynametric measurement of grip strength, with comparison to prevailing strength of peer group. An excellent format is shown in Figure 3-2.

If after examination subsequent consultation is necessary, it should be readily available. Most injuries and problems that occur are of the musculoskeletal system [6]. This area needs special emphasis and can produce a significant yield [3]. Each individual should be examined for specific joint function, range-of-motion (ROM), and presence of pain. Specific emphasis on the ankle and knee is important because of the high instance of injury to these particular joints. Posture and evaluation of the spine may uncover previously unknown scoliosis or leg-length discrepancy. A comprehensive musculoskeletal exam is included in Figure 3-3.

DISPOSITION

After the history and physical examination have been reviewed, the physician must make a decision to

Not allow participation;
Allow participation only in specific sports;
Withhold clearance to participate until additional examinations or tests are completed;

Withold clearance until rehabilitation is complete; or
Allow full, unlimited participation.

CONDITIONS DISQUALIFYING SPORTS PARTICIPATION

Disqualifying conditions have been determined by the American Medical Association [1], and, with some slight modification, are presented here as guidelines. Efforts may be made to overrule a physician's decision by a family and courts. This, however, would leave the responsibility to these parties. A classification of sports is listed in Table 3-1.

1. General conditions
   a. Acute infections (respiratory, genitourinary, infectious mononucleosis, hepatitis, active rheumatic fever, active tuberculosis, boils, furuncles, impetigo)
   b. Herpes simplex (wrestling only)
   c. Obvious physical immaturity in comparison with other competitors (contact and strenuous noncontact sports only)
   d. Obvious growth retardation (contact only)
   e. Bleeding tendencies (contact only)
   f. Diabetes, uncontrolled (all)
   g. Jaundice, all causes (all)
2. Eyes
   a. Absence or loss of function one eye (contact only)
   b. Severe myopia, even if correctable (contact only)
3. Ears: Significant impairment (contact only)
4. Respiratory
   a. Tuberculosis, active (all)
   b. Severe pulmonary insufficiency (all)
5. Cardiovascular
   a. Mitral stenosis, aortic stenosis, aortic insufficiency, coarctation of aorta, cyanotic heart disease, recent carditis of any etiology (all)
   b. Hypertension of organic basis (all)
   c. Previous heart surgery for congenital or acquired heart disease (contact and strenuous noncontact)
6. Liver: Enlarged liver (contact only)
7. Spleen: Enlarged spleen (contact only)
8. Hernia: Femoral or inguinal (contact and strenuous noncontact)
9. Musculoskeletal
   a. Symptomatic abnormalities or inflammation (all)
   b. Functional inadequacy of musculoskeletal system, congenital or acquired, incompatible with the contact or skill demands of the sport (contact and strenuous noncontact)

Table 3-1. Classification of Sports

STRENUOUS

Contact
Footbball
Ice Hockey
Lacrosse (boys)
Rugby
Wrestling

Limited contact
Basketball
Field Hockey
Lacrosse (girls)
Soccer
Volleyball

Noncontact
Crew
Cross-country
Fencing
Gymnastics
Skiing
Swimming
Tennis
Track and field
Water polo

MODERATELY STRENUOUS

Badminton
Baseball (limited contact)
Curling
Golf
Table tennis

NONSTRENUOUS

Archery
Bowling
Riflery

---

10. Neurological
    a. History or symptoms of previous serious head trauma or repeated concussions (contact only)
    b. Convulsive disorder not completely controlled by medication (contact and strenuous noncontact)
    c. Previous surgery on head or spine (contact and strenuous noncontact)
11. Renal
    a. Absence of one kidney (contact only)
    b. Renal disease (all)

12. Genitalia
    a. Absence of one testicle (contact only)
    b. Undescended testicle (contact only)

As noted by Shaffer [9], it is rarely necessary to prohibit nonstrenuous, noncontact sports. Also, acute infections usually only require temporary limitation of activity. Tuberculosis under chemotherapy for two months is not a contraindication to full activity if no other abnormalities are present. Asthma is not a contraindication to participation in sports. The only requirement is that the severity of the condition be ascertained by gradually increasing activity to appearance of respiratory symptoms. Proteinuria in an apparently well child is not a reason for arbitrary disqualification from strenuous sports. Transient proteinuria may occur in any child after vigorous activity [6].

After disposition has been determined, with the results explained to the child athlete, all forms should be signed and dated. All forms should be in triplicate with one copy for school records, a copy for physician records, and a copy for parents [11].

ON-THE-FIELD INJURIES

The physician covering athletic activities has to be prepared to deal with acute injuries; be able to take action quickly should a life-threatening emergency arise; and be able to determine if and when an injured athlete may return to play.

This requires preplanning and a working knowledge of the common athletic injuries, of the indications for removal from play, and of the indications for hospitalization and observation. He or she must have a good working relationship with trainers and equipment managers, and have ready access to ancillary help and expert consultation.

PREPLANNING

The physician must establish the fact that he or she is in charge of all medical matters and makes all decisions regarding the fitness of players before the season begins. The physician must arrange his or her schedule so as to be available for all games throughout the season. He or she should have a working knowledge of suitable standards for equipment, uniforms, and playing fields. With the aid of trainers and coaches, inspection should be undertaken of all equipment, uniforms, and playing fields and when necessary they should be brought up to acceptable standards. Arrangements should be made for a quiet, well-lighted room as close as possible to playing and practice fields with adequate examining, first-aid, and minor treatment equipment.

Communication equipment should be established. Ideally, a telephone would be located on the sidelines to give the physician direct communication with an emergency facility. If no sideline phone is available, a good substitute is a phone in a lock box located nearby, with a key to be issued to appropriate persons. If neither is available, a dime taped inside of the athletic trainer's bag should be common emergency equipment [7].

Arrangements for transportation of an injured player from the field to the sidelines should be made, with a stretcher and if possible a wheeled litter. If the community has an established emergency squad, arrangements should be made to have them present on game days. If an ambulance or other emergency vehicle cannot be used, then a teacher or spectator with a station wagon should be designated the emergency driver. However, this is the least desirable alternative. Finally, arrangements should be made for prompt specialty consultation service throughout the season and backup coverage by a colleague, resident, school nurse, or trainer when necessary.

GAME PROTOCOL

The physician should develop a game-day routine that best utilizes his or her time and the players' time [8]. Arrival should be one hour before game time to make or participate in last-minute decisions regarding players, equipment, playing fields, and even weather.

When a player is down, the physician should go onto the field. He or she is responsible and by far is the best-fitted person present to decide whether the injured player should walk or be carried upright or on a stretcher to the examining room, and to immediately initiate consultation, further evaluation, or definitive treatment, or return the player to the game. He or she should inform the coach as soon as the diagnosis and decision are made. A backup (colleague, resident, etc.) takes the physician's place on the sidelines when he or she is off the field.

At the halftime break the physician personally checks all players for possible concealed injuries and reports any such injuries to the coach. After the game, all injuries, major and minor, are reviewed; crutches, splints, and dressings are checked; parents or guardians are informed; and a written record of every injury is made. The day after the game all injuries should again be reviewed, with final diagnosis and prognosis made. The coach should be informed of all the physician's findings and follow-up notes written.

Criteria for removal from play and for hospital evaluation have been published in the literature [4]. The following are the most widely agreed upon set of such criteria.

A. Criteria for Removal from Play
  1. Eye injury
     a. Blunt trauma
     b. Visual difficulty

    c. Laceration

    d. Obvious deformity

2. Head injury

    a. Loss of consciousness

    b. Disturbed sensorium

    c. Seeing stars or colors

    d. Dizziness

    e. Auditory hallucinations

    f. Nausea

    g. Vomitting

    h. Lethargy

    i. Severe headache

    j. Rising blood pressure

    k. Diminishing pulse

    l. Disturbed smell

    m. Amnesia

    n. Hyperirritability

    o. Large contusion

    p. Open wounds

    q. Unequal pupils

    r. Leakage of cerebrospinal fluid or blood from ears or nose

    s. Numbness of one side of body

3. Neck or spine

    a. Obvious deformity

    b. Weakness of extremity

    c. Loss of motion

    d. Loss of sensation or paresthesia

    e. Localized cervical tenderness

4. Shoulders or extremities

    a. Obvious deformity

    b. Crepitus

    c. Loss of range of motion and loss of sensation

    d. Effusion pain on use

    e. Unstable joints

    f. Open wounds

    g. Significant tenderness

    h. Significant swelling

5. Abdomen

    a. Dizziness or syncope

    b. Nausea

    c. Persisting pallor

    d. Vomiting

    e. History of infectious mononucleosis

    f. Abnormal thirst

    g. Muscle guarding

    h. Localized tenderness

        i. Shoulder pain
        j. Distention
        k. Rapid pulse
        l. Clamminess or sweating

B. General Criteria for Hospital Evaluation
   1. Loss of consciousness for 10 seconds or longer
   2. Drowsiness or stuporous state
   3. Disorientation; retrograde amnesia
   4. Persistent vomiting
   5. Unequal pupils
   6. Battle's sign; ecchymosis over mastoid bone
   7. Leakage of cerebrospinal fluid from nose or ears
   8. Hemorrhage in retina or behind tympanic membrane
   9. Skull fracture
  10. Seizure

Normal activity within a few minutes after the injury is a good sign that the athlete is not seriously injured, but all athletes sustaining a head injury should be kept out of competition until completely asymptomatic.

COMMON ATHLETIC INJURIES

Sprains and strains, contusions, fractures, lacerations, concussion, eye injuries, abdominal trauma, heat-related disorders, and cold injuries compose the majority of injuries seen on the playing field. The first-aid measures for each will be presented.

SPRAINS AND STRAINS

Sprains are partial or complete rupture of ligamentous tissue. Strains are stretch injuries to the musculotendinous unit. Sprains and strains are graded first-degree, or mild, where there is pain but the tissues have not been stretched enough to produce hemorrhage. These injuries are usually not serious enough to stop competition, and when pain subsides, the athlete can usually continue. Swelling may develop later and should be treated with ice, compression, and elevation. The athlete should be restricted from play, however, if unable to maintain an adequate skill level.

Second-degree, or moderate, injuries range from minor tears to almost complete disruption of the tissue. There usually is immediate swelling and pain with decreased function. The athlete with lesser injury may be able to continue play with support to the area, but when more severe, ice, compression, elevation, splinting, and evaluation by a specialist should be the course of treatment.

Third-degree, or severe, injuries involve complete disruption of one or more ligaments or the musculotendinous unit itself. Pain is immediate but may subside. Since the structures are torn through, none of the pain fibers are being stretched. Swelling may be minimal since hemorrhage can extravasate out of the area into the soft tissue. Consequently, the most severe injuries may produce the least symptoms. It is for this reason that the physician must examine all injuries on the field to determine instability from torn ligaments or loss of function from musculotendinous disruptions. When testing the joint for instability it is imperative the physician remember that he is dealing with a growing child and excessive motion may be the result of opening at a growth center rather than disrupted ligaments [7]. If after examination the physician suspects a severe injury, the player should be assisted from the playing field with the injured extremity protected during transfer. X-ray examination of the injured area under stress should be done to demonstrate the problem.

CONTUSIONS

Contusions may be so slight as to go unnoticed until hours or days later, or so severe as to cause gross swelling, loss of function, and pain. A large contusion to the thigh, for example, can cause gross swelling and should be treated with ice, compression, elevation, and early range-of-motion exercises when tolerated. A contusion to the ear may cause hemorrhage under the skin that can progress to fibrosis and a "cauliflower ear." This hematoma should be aspirated sterilely in the first week after injury, with pressure applied to the area. Once normal contours are attained the auricle should be packed with colloidin-soaked cotton or casted with dental plaster for a few days. Ear protectors or padding in the helmet should be used to prevent reinjury [7]. Contusion to the nose may cause a fracture. Digital compression of the septum with the athlete being slightly forward will control hemorrhage and allow breathing through the mouth.

Male genitalia may be traumatized. Ice should be applied to decrease swelling, but if swelling is severe, it should be evaluated by a specialist. A cup protector should be used in any future play. (See Chapter 2.)

FRACTURES

Any blunt trauma that is sufficient to cause a large hematoma may cause a fracture. If there is suspicion of a fracture of an extremity, the limb should be splinted before the athlete is moved. The splint should include the joint above and below the injury. Do not attempt to reduce dislocations. Check peripheral pulses, and if there is an open wound, cover it with a sterile dressing and transport the player to a hospital as soon as possible. Obtain appropriate x-rays and studies at the medical facility [4]. (See Chapter 2. Spinal fractures will be discussed in Chapter 6.)

LACERATIONS

Lacerations, if small, can be managed quite well with tape sutures for the duration of the game. Final repair can be instituted later [7]. Care of larger open wounds should control hemorrhage and decrease bacterial contamination. The wound should be covered with a sterile dressing after the extent of injury is known and the player transferred to a medical facility for definitive treatment. (See Chapter 2.)

CONCUSSION

On-the-field treatment of concussion poses a worrisome problem for the physician. The criteria for removal from play and hospital observation have already been mentioned. Concussions are classified in three ways: first degree, mild, when the athlete is confused, dazed, and may have retrograde amnesia; second degree, moderate, concussions in which unconsciousness occurs for 3 to 4 minutes; and third degree, severe, concussions in which the athlete is unconscious for 5 minutes or longer [7].

Any concussion should end play for that day. When the physician encounters a down player he should assume a cervical fracture until proven otherwise [4, 7]. Check breathing and pulse. (Emergency treatment is discussed in detail in Chapter 2.) If pulse and respiration are normal, wait for consciousness to return, evaluate for orientation, and keep the player still and quiet. A cervical fracture can be ruled out by asking about pain and paresthesia; determine motor power and sensation in extremities and palpate the cervical area. If all is normal proceed to treat the head injury.

Wait until the player is ready to move and assist him to a sitting position. If he is able to sit up, assist him to a kneeling position. When he is able, have the athlete stand and when sure he or she can walk, assist him or her to the sidelines, observing carefully the player's progress. If the athlete cannot progress to walking, call for a stretcher or litter [7]. (See Chapter 2.)

EYE INJURIES

Injury to an eye is a frequent kind of trauma. Remember there is always a chance of intracranial injury by a penetrating foreign body [4]. Do not force eyelids open on the field; treat with ice and compressions for 15-minute intervals, hourly. If visual difficulty is present, keep the athlete lying down and quiet. The eye should never be rubbed. A foreign body can be removed by pulling the upper lid down over the lower lid and pouring warm water over the eyeball. The eye should be bandaged shut and evaluated by a specialist in the appropriate setting.

ABDOMINAL TRAUMA

Abdominal trauma can be life-threatening. The physician should inspect the abdomen for bruises, palpate for tenderness, observe the athlete for muscular guarding, pallor, difficulty breathing, nausea, vomiting, and evidence of fractured ribs. If these signs are present, the player should be taken to the nearest medical facility and worked up [4]. (See Chapter 2.)

HEAT-RELATED DISORDERS

Heat exhaustion and heat stroke are seen during warm temperatures and often confused. Heat exhaustion is due to dehydration and salt loss; the athlete will be cool and moist with a normal temperature. Treatment should include hydration, correction of salt loss, and rest in a cool location with clothing loosened.

Heat stroke is caused by a disruption of the body's thermoregulatory mechanism. The athlete is hot, dry, and red, with a high fever. The athlete must be rapidly cooled with immersion, cool towels, and fanning. He then should be admitted to the hospital and observed [4, 7].

COLD INJURIES

Frostbite has been classified in three stages [4]. First stage, freezing; second stage, freezing with blistering and peeling; third stage, freezing with tissue necrosis. Minor frostbite can be treated with rewarming in a heated room or immersion in warm water. The athlete should avoid trauma and avoid refreezing. Second and third stage frostbite cases should be admitted to the hospital and treated for possible infection or thrombosis.

REFERENCES

1. A Guide for Medical Evaluation of Candidates for School Sports. Chicago: American Medical Association, 1976.
2. Emans, S. J. H., and Goldstein, D. P. *Pediatric and Adolescent Gynecology* (2nd ed.) Boston: Little, Brown, 1982.
3. Goldberg, B., et al. The pre-participation sports assessment—an objective evaluation. *Pediatrics* 66:736, 1980.
4. Greensher, J., Mofenson, H. C., and Merlis, N. J. First aid for school athletic emergencies. *New York J. Med.* 79:1058, 1979.
5. Lonstein, J. E., et al. School screening for the early detection of spinal deformities. *Minn. Med.* 59:51, 1976.
6. Marshall, J. L., and Tischler, H. M. Screening for sports guidelines. *New York J. Med.* 78:243, 1978.
7. Molacrea, R. F. Injuries on the field: The pediatrician as team physician. *Pediatr. Ann.* 7:10, 1978.

8. On Field Management of Athletic Injuries. University of Hawaii, Sports Medicine Course, March 8, 1979.
9. Shaffer, T. E.   The health examination for participation in sports. *Pediatr. Ann.* 7:10, 1978.
10. Strong, W. B., and Alpert, B. S.   The Child with Heart Disease: Play, Recreation and Sports. *Curr. Probl. Pediatr.* 13:2, 1982.
11. The Preseason Physical Exam.   American College of Sports Medicine, 1974.

4. Upper Extremity Injuries in Sports

John B. Emans

APPROACH TO UPPER EXTREMITY INJURIES

Accurate assessment of upper extremity injuries will return the athlete to participation without needless delay and will minimize long-term disability. Many potentially disabling injuries in an upper extremity initially appear minor and are often undertreated. Recognition of the potentially serious upper extremity injury requires careful examination and an awareness of the potential for long-term problems from certain injuries.

In the upper extremity as in all sports-related injuries, it is helpful to distinguish between "macrotrauma" and overuse syndromes of "repetitive microtrauma." Chapter 1 discusses this distinction. Some injuries involve a combination of repetitive microtrauma and a single macrotrauma *Referred pain* is common in the upper extremity and potentially confusing. Vague upper extremity pain with no positive physical findings in the area of pain should always lead to the search for referred pain.

HAND INJURIES

Significant hand injuries that are easily undertreated or overlooked are:

Gamekeeper's thumb (rupture of the ulnar collateral ligament metacarpal phalangeal [MP] joint of thumb)
Flexor tendon rupture
Mallet "baseball" finger (rupture of the terminal extensor tendon)
Boutonniere deformity (rupture of the central slip extensor tendon)
Bennett's fracture of thumb (unstable fracture-dislocation of the carpometacarpal [CM] joint of thumb)

These injuries are commonly underdiagnosed, but remaining alert to their significance will lead to appropriate treatment. These are discussed individually under the appropriate subheadings of "Fractures," "Tendon ruptures," or "Sprains."

EXAMINATION OF THE INJURED HAND

Proper examination of the injured hand requires a search for deformity, limitation of motion, tenderness, instability, and an assessment of nerve and tendon function. The following steps are suggested in the examination of a closed or open injury of the hand.

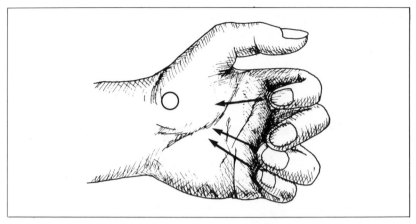

Figure 4-1. Malalignment of long finger associated with a fracture. When partially clenched, all fingers should point approximately to the base of the thenar eminence. Malalignment suggests malrotation of a metacarpal or phalangeal fracture.

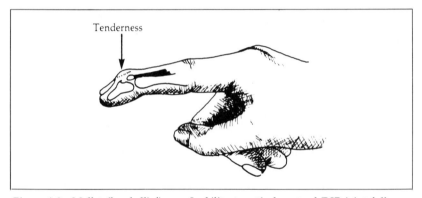

Figure 4-2. Mallet (baseball) finger. Inability to actively extend DIP joint fully because of extensor tendon rupture.

Deformity

Look for malalignment, malrotation, or obvious deformity. Is the posture of the fingers normal? If not, this may signify a tendon rupture (Figures 4-1, 4-2, 4-3).

Tenderness

Can the patient's tenderness be localized to a limited bony, ligamentous, or muscular area? Localized tenderness will universally lead to a diagnosis.

Motion

Is there restriction of motion in a digit; if so, is it localized to one joint? Is it a restriction in active motion or passive motion or both?

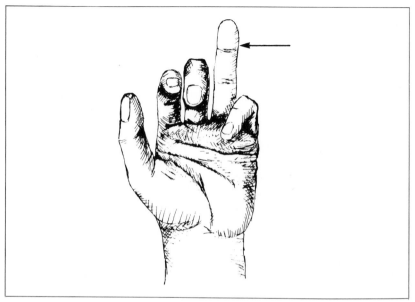

Figure 4-3. Injury of flexor tendon. Abnormal posturing of ring finger at rest (arrow) suggests rupture of flexor tendon.

Instability

Is there any instability relating to the area of tenderness? Joints should be gently tested for instability.

Nerve Function

Injured areas should be tested for sensation. Function of the three major nerves in the hand should be tested individually (Figures 4-4, 4-5).

Tendon Function

Injured digits should be checked carefully for tendon function of the extensor apparatus and both flexor tendons (Figures 4-6, 4-7).

CONTUSIONS

Contusions occur frequently in the hand, both in upper extremity sports and those not specifically involving the upper extremities. The appropriate treatment of simple contusions is (1) elevation to minimize the bleeding and swelling that occur subsequent to the injury, (2) gentle compression, and (3) ice. Contusions are self-limiting and an athlete may be returned to participation as soon as symptoms permit. Temporary padding taped over the contusion may help. Contusions with no underlying bony injuries are distinguished by the lack of bone tenderness or pain on joint motion. An x-ray may be necessary to ensure that no fracture lies beneath the contusion.

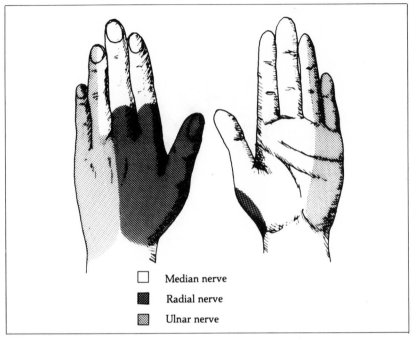

Figure 4-4. Typical sensory distribution in the hand.

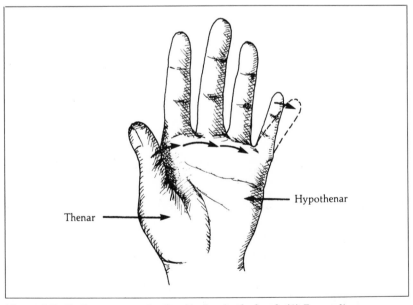

Figure 4-5. Testing nerve-motor functioning in the hand. (1) For median nerve—
test ability of thenar muscles to bring thumb away from palm against resistance.
(2) For ulnar nerve—test ability of hypothenar muscles to abduct fifth finger
against resistance.

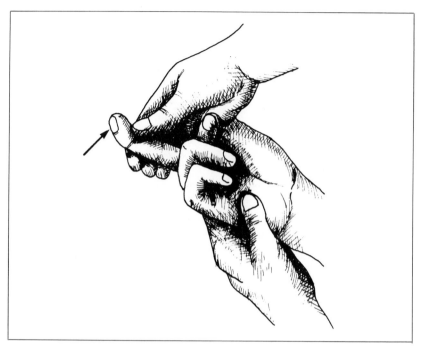

Figure 4-6. Testing flexor digitorum profundus tendon. If DIP joint can be actively flexed while PIP joint is stabilized, profundus tendon has not been severed.

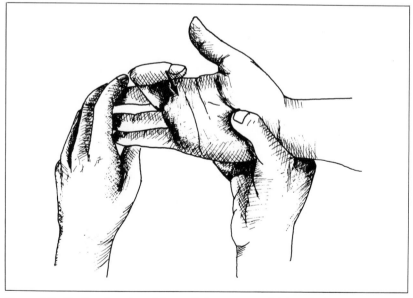

Figure 4-7. Testing function of flexor digitorum superficialis. If PIP joint can be actively flexed whil adjacent fingers are held completely extended, sublimis tendon is intact.

A crushing injury of the hand, such as sometimes caused by baseball or football cleats, although technically a contusion, may result in massive swelling requiring much more aggressive splinting and elevation and occasionally surgical decompression. The rapid appearance of swelling after a crushing injury should suggest this possibility and the hand should be splinted and maximally elevated while seeking specialized care.

LACERATIONS

Initially, when examining a laceration, one should search for nerve or tendon injury as well as underlying fracture or instability.

The profusely bleeding hand laceration naturally focuses the examiner's attention on the skin. A major laceration or the most innocuous appearing puncture wound may mask major nerve and tendon injury. In the rush to treat the laceration these are easily overlooked but are of greater significance than the actual laceration. A careful sensory examination and tendon examination based on a knowledge of potentially injured structures must always be performed for even the most minor looking laceration. Figures 4-4 to 4-7 review sensory examination and motor examination, and indicate the method for examining for tendon injury. Pain on moving a joint or tendon remote from the laceration may indicate a partial tendon laceration and should be referred immediately. Techniques for the primary repair of nerve lacerations and the primary suture of lacerated tendons in the hand have improved tremendously. In a clean, fresh wound some surgeons now repair tendons primarily wherever possible. Thus, the practice of treating the skin laceration and referring the patient for later tendon repair should, wherever possible, be replaced by emergency referral to the appropriate specialist.

Treating the Laceration

Consider obtaining an x-ray if a foreign body is remotely possible. An imbedded piece of glass or stone from a fall on the ground or a piece of tooth from a blow may be revealed in this manner. Assess the cleanliness of the wound. Where there is obvious dirt or debris in the wound or the injury is a laceration incurred by contact with a tooth, the wound should rarely be closed primarily. Most lacerations incurred in the course of athletics are relatively dirty because of playing field conditions, equipment, or contact with other competitors. Much more harm is caused by the infection resulting from a primarily closed dirty wound than from the larger scar resulting from delayed closure.

Cleansing the Wound and Debridement

Proper cleansing is far more important than suture technique. Cleansing of lacerations is often facilitated by a small amount of Xylocaine injected in the wound edges. This enables one to scrub the skin adjacent to the wound and irrigate the depths of the wound. In some wounds this is best accomplished by scrubbing the hand under running water with a surgeon's preoperative sponge brush. The depths of the wound can be irrigated with saline from a syringe without a needle and the depths of the wound investigated for any debris.

Closure of the Wound

If conditions are optimal, close the wound with interrupted, loosely opposed, monofilament, nonabsorbable sutures such as 4–0 nylon. A tightly closed wound leads to necrosis of the skin edges and will not allow escape of blood or any residual contamination. The number of stitches should be kept to a minimum. "Steri-strips" applied with benzoin are a reasonable solution in many locations. When in doubt, pack the wound open with gauze and plan a delayed primary closure 48 hours later or allow the wound to heal spontaneously.

Antibiotics

Prophylactic antibiotics have no role in routine lacerations. They will not compensate for inadequate cleansing or inappropriate closure. Some surgeons do advocate their use routinely for major human bites.

Tetanus

The child's immunization status should be ascertained and tetanus toxoid given if appropriate.

Return to Participation

If the laceration can be reasonably protected with a reinforced dressing, the athlete may return to participation immediately. If the sport requires immersion, repeated pressure on the laceration, or contact with a very contaminated area, early healing of the wound (2–5 days) should be allowed first.

PUNCTURE WOUNDS

Although outwardly innocuous, puncture wounds may conceal significant nerve or tendon injury. The same search for associated injuries should be made as in a laceration. The potential for accumulation of hematoma and the difficulty in adequately cleansing puncture wounds greatly increase the potential for infection. If a puncture wound appears deep or was caused by a potentially dirty object, it is wiser to make a small incision enlarging the puncture wound and carry out adequate irrigation, debridement, and exploration of the wound as with a larger laceration. Puncture wounds should be observed more frequently for signs of infection than a routine laceration. Puncture wounds that overlie a joint should be assumed to penetrate the joint and referred for treatment.

SPRAINS AND LIGAMENT RUPTURES

The spectrum of ligament injury in the hand ranges from a minor sprain in which a ligament is stretched slightly beyond its normal excursion, to a complete ligament rupture in which the substance of the ligament is torn or its attachment to bone is avulsed. Accurate assessment of these injuries depends upon localizing the ligament tenderness as accurately as possible and assessing the stability of the joint involved. Significant ligament injuries are easily overlooked in the hand, particularly about the PIP joints. An x-ray is suggested for all "sprains."

Distal Interphalangeal (DIP) Sprains

DIP joint sprains are unusual and should be distinguished from extensor tendon injuries (see mallet finger below), flexor profundis tendon avulsion (see below), and fractures.

Proximal Interphalangeal (PIP) Joint Sprains

Hyperextension injuries to the PIP joint are common in many sports and are characterized by swelling, tenderness over the volar aspect of the PIP joint, and pain on hyperextension. These involve injury to the volar plate, a fibrocartilaginous structure that covers the volar aspect of the PIP joint. With a lateral force, the ulnar or radial collateral ligaments of the PIP joint may be sprained and may actually be ruptured. In the case of a collateral ligament rupture, tenderness will be localized to the lateral side of the joint and pain produced on stressing the ligament with a lateral force. If instability of the joint is sensed during this testing, this may signify complete rupture. If tenderness is greatest on the dorsum of the PIP joint, damage to the central slip of the extensor tendon should be suspected. This is described below under Boutonniere Deformity. Simple sprains of the PIP joint without instability can be treated symptomatically with a short splint in 45 degrees of flexion immobilizing just the PIP joint for 7 to 10 days. This type of splint can often be incorporated in a padded dressing consisting of multiple layers of tape, and, if taped to an adjacent finger for additional support, will usually allow the athlete to participate in most sports. PIP joint sprains with instability or a suspected Boutonniere deformity should be referred for treatment. A sprain in which full joint motion is not possible may be due to an underlying fracture or ligament entrapment and should be referred.

Metacarpal Phalangeal (MP) Joint Sprains

Excessive forces applied to the MP joint of the fingers can result in strains of the volar plate characterized by tenderness on the volar aspect of the MP joint and pain on hyperextension. Excessive force in a lateral direction can strain or rupture the collateral ligaments of the MP joint. As in PIP joint injuries, a search should be made for medial and lateral instability by stressing the finger. Volar tenderness suggests a volar plate injury, and radial or ulnar tenderness signifies collateral ligament injury. A splint incorporating the proximal phalanx and metacarpal in a position of 60 to 90 degrees of MP flexion for 7 to 10 days is adequate treatment for simple MP joint sprains. Sprains with instability or a block to full motion should be referred for treatment.

Sprains of the MP Joint of the Thumb

The MP joint of the thumb is particularly susceptible to sprain because of its isolated position. A fall on the outstretched and abducted thumb, an attempt to block a maneuver with the outstretched hand, and a fall on a hand fixed by a ski pole strap are common mechanisms for injury to the thumb MP joint. Sprains to this joint are characterized by swelling and fairly localized tenderness. A hyperextension injury will usually produce stretching of the volar structures and volar tenderness. An abducting injury will stress the radial collateral ligaments and produce tenderness on the radial aspect of the joint. The most common potentially disabling injury, however, is the "gamekeeper's thumb," which is a sprain of the ulnar collateral ligaments of the thumb MP joint produced by hyperabducting the MP joint (Figure 4-8). This is accompanied by swelling and tenderness over the ulnar aspect of the joint. Since motion of the MP joint may not be restricted and initial function may be minimally impaired, this potentially significant injury is easily missed. A partial sprain of the MP joint ulnar collateral ligaments should be treated with seven to ten days of splinting of the MP joint alone. However, a sprain of the ulnar collateral ligament that is accompanied by instability in most cases should be treated oper-

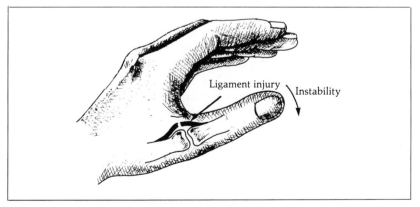

Figure 4-8. Gamekeeper's thumb (rupture of ulnar collateral ligament of the thumb) results in lateral instability of the MP joint.

atively. The important distinction between a partial and complete tear of the ulnar collateral ligament is made by flexing the thumb MP joint about 20 degrees and abducting the thumb in a radialward direction. This sometimes requires local anesthesia to overcome the patient's discomfort. Mobility in excess of the opposite normal thumb should lead to the diagnosis of a rupture of the ulnar collateral ligament and the patient should be referred immediately. The term *gamekeeper's thumb* stems from the chronic instability noted in game wardens from their method of killing fowl. The untreated complete ulnar collateral ligament rupture in many cases leads to the same sort of instability and can be significantly disabling. A stable ulnar collateral ligament is required for a strong pinch between the thumb and adjacent fingers. Following a simple sprain of the MP joint of the thumb, the thumb can be protected for several weeks in most athletes by providing a web of taping between the thumb and base of the index finger or palm, thus preventing a repeat abduction injury of the metacarpal phalangeal joint.

CM Joint of the Thumb

Simple sprains of the carpometacarpal joint of the thumb occur less frequently than those of the MP joint and are usually not accompanied by instability. A search should be made for a fracture dislocation of the carpometacarpal joint since this too will produce pain and swelling in the region of the CM joint and is of much greater significance. Simple sprains of this joint can be treated nonspecifically either by splinting the base of the thumb or by taping for support.

DISLOCATIONS OF THE FINGERS

Dislocations of the fingers of athletes are common and carry a number of euphemistic names such as "coach's finger," "football finger," or "jammed finger." For the tightly constrained joints of the fingers and thumb to dislocate, significant stretching and/or rupture of one or more ligamentous or capsular structures usually must occur. Dislocations in which the displacement has occurred laterally usually involve complete rupture of a collateral ligament. Dislocations in which the distal bone has been displaced volarward often rupture the insertion of the extensor mechanism at the joint, and dislocations with the distal bone displacing dorsally usually rupture the volar plate and may occasionally involve damage to a flexor tendon. Many coaches, trainers, and well-meaning bystanders will reduce the dislocation for an injured athlete, and if already reduced, an attempt should be made to ascertain in which direction the dislocation occurred.

Dislocations require an x-ray before reduction to confirm the direction of the dislocation and assure that no major fracture accompanies the dislocation. Sensation should be checked and insofar as possible tendon function assessed. With the aid of a digital nerve block at the base of the finger, an ulnar nerve block at the elbow, a median nerve block at the wrist, or if necessary with no anesthesia, most digital dislocations can be easily reduced with simple longitudinal traction.

Occasionally irreducible dislocations of the MP joint or PIP joint occur and unreasonable force should not be applied. Reduction should be confirmed by an x-ray, the collateral ligaments tested for stability, and a careful check of tendon function made after relocation. It is possible that a portion of the joint capsule can be trapped within the relocated joint and the injured joint should move through a full arc of passive motion with the aid of local anesthesia. Lack of full passive motion, instability of the collateral ligament, or tendency for the joint to re-dislocate should be grounds for referral.

If the dislocation is stable and the above criteria are met, most dislocations can then be easily treated with splinting at 45 degrees of flexion for the PIP joints and 60 to 90 degrees of flexion for the MP joints of the finger for 10 days. Considerable stiffness will be encountered after this and a return to participation may have to be delayed until a functional arc of motion is achieved. Almost all dislocations of the MP and CM joint of the thumb are unstable and should be referred.

TENDON INJURIES

The flexor and extensor tendon mechanisms are relatively resistant to injury, particularly in the youthful athlete where epiphyseal fractures are more common. Prompt recognition of tendon disruptions by the primary physician is crucial.

Flexor Tendon Injuries

A laceration of the flexor tendons should be suspected in any laceration of the volar aspect of the fingers, hand, wrist, or distal forearm. This can be ruled in or out only by a careful physical examination. Function of the flexor profundus and the flexor sublimis must be delineated in each finger (see Figures 4-3, 4-6, 4-7). Lacerated flexor tendons or suspected tendon laceration should be dressed and referred immediately.

Flexor tendon rupture also occurs in the absence of penetrating injury. This occurs most commonly in football when the jersey that a tackler's hands are forcibly grasping is suddenly pulled away. This results in forcible extension of the fingers while the flexor mechanism is under maximum contraction. The flexor profundus tendon can then rupture at the level of its insertion or more proximally. This is accompanied by pain and swelling along the tendon sheath, mild restriction of motion only, and usually abonormal posturing of the DIP joint. A careful test of flexor digitorum profundus and sublimis function will demonstrate disruption of the tendon. This should be splinted in flexion at the wrist and finger and referred immediately since further contraction of the muscle belly may pull the proximal tendon fragment farther away from the site of rupture.

Extensor Tendon Ruptures

The extensor mechanism can be lacerated at any level along the dorsum of the wrist, hand, and finger. Often such lacerations are trivial. Closed injuries to the extensor mechanism are common.

"Mallet finger" ("baseball finger"; see Figure 4-2) occurs when the common extensor insertion into the dorsum of the distal phalanx is disrupted. Most commonly this occurs when the end of the finger is struck directly by a ball or other object forcing it into hyperflexion. If the extensor mechanism is contracting at that moment, the common insertion into the dorsum of the distal phalanx will be avulsed or avulsed with a small fragment of bone. This is a relatively painless injury and does not result in any immediate disability. Often it goes unrecognized for several days and finally presents when the patient notices the end of the finger beginning to droop. Left untreated, the finger will continue to droop. Diagnosis is easily made by testing the range of active extension of the DIP joint, which will be greatly lacking in comparison to adjacent fingers. The treatment is almost always closed splinting of the DIP joint in hyperextension for 6 to 8 weeks. During the early stages of this splinting care must be taken never to allow the DIP joint to fall into flexion. Usually this can be accomplished by splinting the joint alone. Some surgeons prefer also to splint the PIP joint in flexion. Mallet finger deformities are best splinted in hyperextension and referred on a nonemergency basis to an orthopedic or hand surgeon for supervision of the prolonged splinting required.

Boutonniere Deformity

The Boutonniere deformity (Figure 4-9) occurs after rupture of the central extensor slip attaching to the dorsum of the base of the middle phalanx. This may occur as part of a PIP joint sprain or dislocation, a minor laceration over the dorsum of the proximal phalanx or PIP joint, or as an isolated injury in which the PIP joint is suddenly hyperflexed while the extensor mechanism is taut. Minimal pain and swelling are involved, but if it is left untreated, a progressive deformity of flexion at the PIP joint and hyperextension at the DIP joint will develop. A potential Boutonniere deformity should be suspected in every PIP joint sprain in which there is some degree of dorsal joint tenderness. If the patient is unable to actively extend the PIP joint to neutral, then this injury must be considered. Treatment of the Boutonniere deformity in its late stages is controversial. In its early stages it can be treated by splinting the PIP joint in full extension. Because

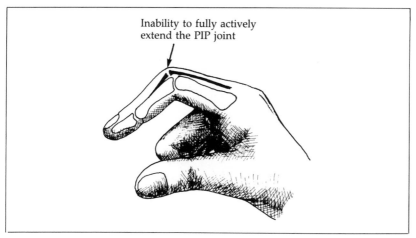

Inability to fully actively
extend the PIP joint

Figure 4-9. Boutonniere deformity. Rupture of the central extensor tendon slip at the PIP joint.

of the potential for late deformity this injury should be referred to a knowledgeable hand or orthopedic surgeon.

FRACTURES

Fractures of the bones of the hand are perhaps the most common significant hand injury in athletes. Almost all can be treated easily, if properly diagnosed, but if allowed to remain in lateral angulation, malrotation or, if joint surfaces are involved, a serious cosmetic or functional deficit may result. The primary physician should attempt to identify the injury and determine its seriousness. Simple well-aligned fractures can be treated with a minimum of experience. Most crucial, however, is the recognition that the fracture is malaligned or malrotated. X-rays alone are often deceiving in that the severely mal-rotated fracture may look nicely aligned on x-ray. Emphasis should, therefore, be placed on clinical examination or alignment of the injured bones (see Figure 4-1).

Phalangeal Fractures

Phalangeal fractures are common and if undisplaced and not associated with an open wound, tendon injury, malrotation, or visible deformity, can easily be treated by the nonorthopedist. Fractures that are displaced, enter the joint, or are associated with instability, as well as those that remain malrotated, should be referred. The simple nondisplaced phalangeal fracture should be immobilized in plaster or aluminum splint with the MP joint in 60 to 90 degrees of flexion and the PIP joint in 45 degrees of flexion until stability has been achieved. This requires about 10 days to 2 weeks in most children. Thereafter the simple phalangeal fracture can be immobilized until solidly healed (about 4 to 6 weeks by taping the injured finger to the adjacent finger or fingers).

Epiphyseal Fractures

Fractures of this type that fulfill the same criteria as phalangeal fractures can be treated in a like fashion. Because the bone adjacent to the epiphysis heals rapidly the total period of immobilization can be somewhat less than that for phalangeal fractures.

Joint Fractures

Joint fractures should be referred even though small in size. Joint fractures may result in lasting incongruity of the joint surface or, as in the case of the dorsal lip fracture at the base of the proximal end of the distal phalanx, may signify tendon avulsion.

Metacarpal Fractures

These are another type of common fracture, particularly those of the fourth and fifth metacarpals. In a growing child considerable angulation can be accepted because of remodeling potential, but no malrotation is tolerated (see Figure 4-1). The metacarpal shaft fracture or metacarpal neck fracture that is minimally angulated and not displaced and not associated with malrotation can be treated by splinting with plaster for about 10 days to 2 weeks, and then protecting the involved digit by taping to the adjacent digits. If competition is feasible, padding can be added over the fracture itself. Displaced or angulated fractures, those with malrotation, and those in question should be referred.

Bennett's Fracture

This fracture occurs at the base of the thumb CM joint. To the untrained eye this may at first seem an innocuous injury. In this fracture-dislocation, the base of the metacarpal dislocates radially and proximally, leaving behind a small avulsion fracture off the ulnar corner of the metacarpal. All thumb metacarpal fractures passing through the CM joint should be referred for treatment.

WRIST AND FOREARM INJURIES

Significant injuries of the wrist and forearm that are easily overlooked are navicular fractures and intercarpal ligamentous instability.

Most commonly, wrist and forearm injuries occur in a fall on the involved upper extremity, and the diagnosis of a major wrist or forearm fracture is readily apparent. Wrist sprains are relatively uncommon in growing children and less common in adolescents. Tenderness over the carpal bones or radiocarpal joint should make one first suspect a navicular or other carpal fracture and should lead to a careful x-ray search for fracture.

A subluxation of the distal radioulnar joint is not uncommon, occurring often with a fall on the outstretched hand or sometimes in association with a metacarpal or other hand injury. This diagnosis is made by prominence of the distal ulnar styloid relative to the normal side and tenderness over the distal radioulnar articulation. Pronation and supination will be painful, but regular x-rays are normal. Faced with tenderness over the distal radioulnar joint and the possibility of subluxation, a patient should be referred acutely to an orthopedist. Distal radial ulnar dislocation or subluxation is usually treated with a long arm cast in supination.

Significant ruptures of the intercarpal ligaments do occur and are manifested by wrist swelling and tenderness over the carpal bones, particularly on the dorsum. Volar flexion particularly will be uncomfortable. The diagnosis of intercarpal instability is difficult to make even for the orthopedist and requires special x-ray views. The apparent wrist sprain with no visible fracture, tenderness over the carpal bones, and soft tissue swelling, or the wrist sprain in which discomfort persists for more than a week, should suggest a significant intercarpal injury and the possibility of ligamentous instability. The same symptoms with persistent tenderness over the anatomic snuff box should lead to the search for a navicular fracture.

A simple wrist sprain without instability can be treated symptomatically and the athlete's wrist can often be taped and returned to activity as soon as symptoms permit.

EXAMINATION OF THE INJURED WRIST AND FOREARM

The wrist and forearm as a unit are capable of pronation and supination, volar flexion and dorsiflexion, and radial and ulnar deviation. In addition, there are complex motions that occur between the carpal bones in all wrist motions. An assessment of any wrist injury demands examination of the range of motion in all of these directions and comparison with the opposite side. Localization of tenderness or reproduction of symptoms with a particular motion will lead to the appropriate anatomic diagnosis. In the wrist and forearm many structures are crowded together making diagnosis difficult. Tenderness of an overlying tendon can be distinguished from tenderness of underlying bone by motion or stressing the suspected tendon.

FRACTURES

Most wrist and forearm fractures should be readily apparent.

Navicular Fracture

A navicular fracture is often overlooked because it is not associated with major trauma, has minimal swelling, and, at first, minimal disability. Typically it mimics a wrist "sprain" but symptoms persist beyond several days. Untreated navicular fractures often proceed to a nonunion and require secondary surgery. Faced with any wrist injury, the examiner should look for a navicular fracture since the incidence

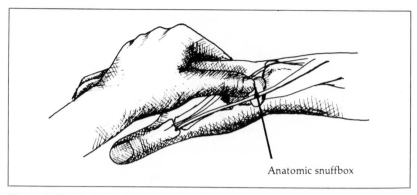

Figure 4-10. *Navicular fracture. Tenderness over the anatomic snuffbox on the radial surface of the hand is seen with a fracture of the carpal navicular.*

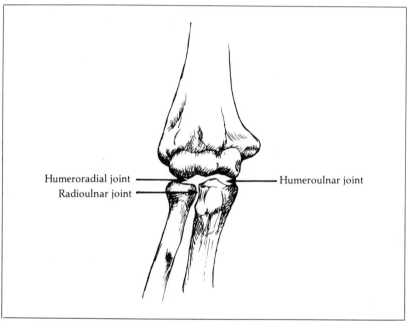

Figure 4-11. *The elbow joint is actually composed of three distinct articulations.*

of nonunion with freshly treated navicular fractures is very low compared with those in which diagnosis has been greatly delayed. Typically, a navicular fracture will exhibit tenderness in the anatomic snuffbox (Figure 4-10) and be associated with pain at the extremes of wrist motion. X-rays, including navicular views, will often be normal at the time of injury, but 10 days to 2 weeks later x-rays should be repeated if snuffbox tenderness was present originally or persists (Figure 4-11). These subsequent x-rays will then reveal the navicular fracture. Standard treatment consists of immobilization in a long thumb spica cast until the fracture has healed, which may be as much as 3 to 4 months, even in a freshly diagnosed fracture.

Buckle Fractures

Buckle fractures of the distal radius and ulna are often missed in children and considered to be sprains. These are nondisplaced fractures, so-named because of a small irregularity of the cortex seen in the A-P view. Although most buckle fractures will proceed uneventfully to union with no treatment, they should be immobilized until healed to prevent a major displaced fracture from occurring at the same site during their healing phase. Since most buckle fractures of the distal radius and ulnar are very stable, children can usually be returned to activity immediately provided the cast is strong enough and adequately padded to prevent injury to other participants. For water sports, a removable cast or waterproof cast can be arranged.

OVERUSE INJURIES

Many upper extremity sports generate overuse injuries in the forearm and wrist. Repetitive weight lifting, pole vaulting, javelin, rowing, and racquet sports all exact their toll in overuse injuries.

Tendinitis

This is easily recognized by tenderness over the course of the tendon often associated with some swelling and a "squeaky" or crepitant feeling on moving the tendon. Although mild increase in temperature may be present, erythema, warmth, or more massive swelling should suggest an infection or the synovitis associated with an acute arthritis. Actual tendon ruptures in the wrist and forearm are unusual in children but the occasional flexor tendon rupture occurring in the digital sheath or palm may manifest as more proximal synovitis.

Digital Extensor Tendon Tenosynovitis

This condition is associated with swelling starting just proximal to the metacarpal heads and extending to the wrist, where the swelling often is constricted by ligaments and then may reappear on the distal forearm.

DeQuervain's Disease

This condition, tenosynovitis of the abductor pollicis longus, is a distinct syndrome consisting of exquisite tenderness and some swelling, usually well localized at the course of these tendons over the radial styloid. Resisted abduction and extension of the thumb reproduce these symptoms or passive adduction and flexion of the thumb associated with ulnar deviation of the wrist exacerbate them.

Flexor Tendon Synovitis

This usually involves all of the tendons passing through the carpal tunnel volarly and is associated with deep tenderness and swelling and pain on resisted flexion of the wrist and fingers. If severe enough this may cause median nerve compromise and the symptoms of medial nerve deficiency seen in adults.

Ganglions

These formations occur frequently on the dorsum of the wrist and attention to their existence is brought about by minor trauma. The localized, firm, nontender characteristics of a ganglion distinguish it from tenosynovitis. Although rare, soft tissue neoplasms may resemble a ganglion. An asymptomatic ganglion needs no specific treatment and is not a contraindication to sporting activities.

ELBOW INJURIES

Most injuries to the elbow are minor and self-limiting and easily treated by the generalist. Most difficulty is encountered distinguishing minor contusions and sprains from the more subtle fractures and joint injuries. Readily apparent fractures and dislocations should be referred immediately for treatment.

ANATOMY

The motions permitted by the normal elbow include a full arc of flexion and extension and almost 180 degrees of pronation and supination. The olecranon glides along the trochlea of the humerus in flexion and extension, and the head of the radius glides along the surface of the humeral capitellum in flexion and extension. Pronation and supination of the forearm are permitted by rotation of the radial head relative to the capitellum and within the constraints of the annular ligament of the proximal radius. In addition the margins of the radial head slide within a corresponding group on the olecranon (see Figure 4-11). There is little tolerance for error in this complex system and little inherent bony stability of the elbow joint. For stability the elbow relies heavily upon ligamentous structures and when subjected to abnormal or repetitive stresses frequently is injured.

RADIOLOGIC ANATOMY

Interpretation of elbow x-rays in the growing child is made difficult by the stepwise appearance of multiple centers of secondary ossification. Longitudinal growth of the lower end of the humerus occurs through an enchondral sequence in the lower humeral epiphyseal plate, but in addition, a traction apophysis at the medial epicondyle and olecranon are present. The secondary center of ossification in the lateral humeral condyle appears later than in the medial humeral condyle. There are also separate centers of ossification for the olecranon and radial head (Figure 4-12).

Since many fractures occur through the cartilaginous growth plates or cartilaginous models of the elbow, it is difficult to see many elbow fractures in the growing child. The so-called fat pad sign (Figure 4-13) is a clue to the presence of intra-articular effusion and its presence in a traumatized elbow should be taken to mean fracture until proven otherwise. Comparison x-rays of the opposite elbow may help delineate a fracture.

EXAMINATION

Examination of the symptomatic elbow should include range of motion in flexion and extension, pronation and supination, a test of active strength through these motions, and a brief examination of distal neurological function to look for median, radial, or ulnar neuropathy. In the traumatized elbow a systemic search for tenderness, including the medial and lateral humeral metaphysis; the medial and lateral epicondyles; the olecranon; and the radial head, radial capitellar, and humeral olecranon joints will often be as helpful as x-rays. Swelling of the elbow after trauma usually means a fracture, especially in the younger child. As mentioned above, the fat pad sign may be positive and traumatized; swollen elbow should be treated as a fracture until proven otherwise by consultation. Applying a varus or valgus stress while flexing and extending or pronating and supinating may reproduce the patient's symptoms or cause locking, particularly if a throwing sport is involved.

FRACTURES

Medial Humeral Epicondyle Fractures

These can occur with relatively minor trauma and are basically avulsion fractures. A sudden throw or twist or fall may result in avulsion of the medial epicondyle by the attached forearm flexor muscle origins. Tenderness and swelling in the medial humerus along with a difference in the x-ray as compared with the opposite side will lead to the appropriate diagnosis. Most of these fractures require open reduction.

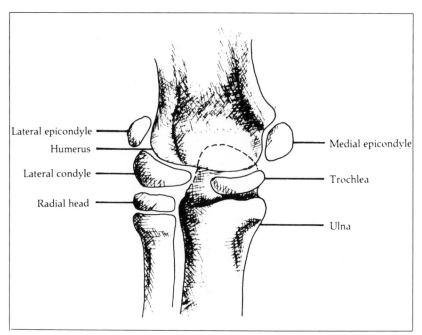

Figure 4-12. Radiologic appearance of growing elbow. Note multiple centers of secondary ossification.

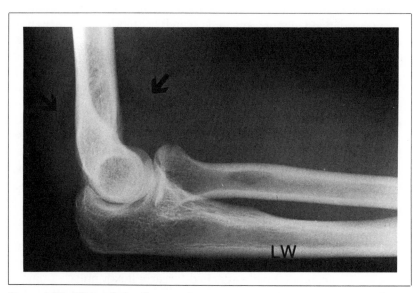

Figure 4-13. "Fat pad sign."

Transcondylar or Supracondylar Fractures

These are usually readily apparent, but in a growing child a wide epiphyseal plate may make diagnosis difficult. Swelling and tenderness at the distal humeral metaphysis should always suggest a nondisplaced transcondylar fracture.

Lateral Humeral Condyle Fractures

These may occur completely through areas of nonossified cartilage and may occur with minimal trauma. Diagnosis is often restricted to lateral tenderness, swelling, restriction of motion, and subtle differences between the x-ray of the affected side and the opposite side. Similarly, fractures of the *radial head* may occur in association with wrist fractures or as isolated injuries. Tenderness over the radial neck and a subtle difference in x-rays will result in the diagnosis.

DISLOCATIONS

Complete elbow dislocations are readily apparent on physical exam and associated with massive swelling and sometimes with neurovascular injury. Transient dislocation or subluxation of the radial head occurs in very young children as "nursemaid's elbow" associated with a pull on the outstretched arm. This is not a common occurrence in the child involved with athletics. If a radiohumeral dislocation is suspected, careful comparison of the alignment on x-ray of the proximal radius with the humeral capitellum will confirm this. Since associated fractures are frequent, ligamentous instability or medial humeral epicondyle fracture not uncommon, and the possibility of Volkmann's ischemia or neurovascular injury high, any elbow dislocation should be referred for treatment even though it may be reduced.

OLECRANON BURSITIS

This condition may mimic significant injury. A direct blow to the olecranon may result in local soft tissue swelling and bleeding or effusion within the olecranon bursa. This swelling is restricted to the olecranon surface of the elbow and not associated with any restriction of motion or bony tenderness. If no fracture is present by x-ray, the olecranon bursitis may be treated symptomatically and protected with elasticized elbow pads or improvised padding taped in place. If associated with signs of infection, this should be aspirated first for a diagnosis under very careful sterile conditions. Open drainage of olecranon bursitis is rarely indicated.

ULNAR NEUROPATHY

The ulnar nerve passes from the medial portion of the arm beneath the medial epicondyle, passing posterior to the axis of flexion in the elbow and thence beneath the flexor muscle mass into the forearm. In its position in the olecranon groove it is exposed to direct trauma (hence the "funny bone") and can be injured by direct blows on the elbow. Sometimes a combination of repetitive elbow movements, repetitive valgus stretch on the elbow, and underlying anatomic abnormality such as constriction of the ulnar nerve, or a valgus deformity in the elbow, may result in chronic ulnar neuropathy. This may be manifested as a weakness of the intrinsic muscles of the hand with wasting of the hypothenar eminence, weakness of the flexor profundus to the fifth and fourth fingers, or as repetitive sensory dysesthesias in the ulnar distribution. Treatment for this varies depending on its etiology, but ulnar neuropathy should be brought to the attention of a specialist.

OVERUSE INJURIES

With the exception of the knee, the elbow is the most commonly encountered site of overuse injuries. Although well suited to a wide range of motion, the elbow seems prone to injury from repetitive stresses. Although with many athletic activities discomfort in the general region of the biceps, triceps, or forearm musculature can be expected, any patient complaining of persistent elbow discomfort after activity has a significant injury. Many of the residua of chronic elbow overuse injuries are not apparent until years later. Thus, a symptomatic elbow should be investigated very carefully until an etiology for the activity-induced discomfort is found. By paying close attention to any elbow symptoms in youth the dreaded residua of elbow injuries can be minimized.

Throwing Injuries

Injuries associated with throwing are encountered in a variety of sports. Maximum velocity is imparted to the thrown object by transferring forward momentum of the body or torque to the thrown object using the arm as a lever arm. Greater speed can be obtained with the arm in a maximally extended position by unwinding the shoulder late, by throwing side-arm, and other maneuvers. The basic throwing position places the elbow under tremendous stress (Figure 4-14).

A valgus force applied to the elbow results in stretching of the medial structures and a compressive force on the lateral structures (Figure 4-15). In baseball this may manifest as chronic medial epicondylitis with overgrowth of the medial epicondyle from chronic traction. Sometimes a sudden avulsion of the previously weakened medial epicondyle occurs with a hard throw. The ulnar collateral ligament of the elbow may be chronically strained with loose body formation beneath the medial epicondyle manifested by persistent medial pain or aching and sometimes by episodes of locking or catching. Chronic compressive forces on the lateral side of the elbow may produce radiohumeral joint degenerative changes, osteochondritis of the capitellum with or with-

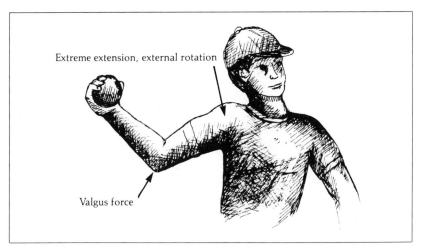

Figure 4-14. Forces on the elbow and shoulder with throwing.

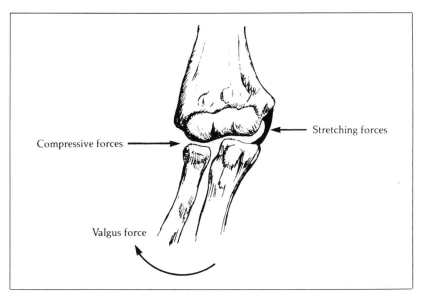

Figure 4-15. At the elbow, lateral compression forces and medial distraction forces result from throwing.

out loose body formation, and, sometimes, growth retardation or angulation of the growing radial head. Common to all of these problems is pain felt in the elbow, restriction of elbow motion compared with normal, or a sense of catching or locking.

Gymnastics

This sport, with its emphasis on repetitive upper extremity activities, may produce a constellation of symptoms similar to throwing injuries. Because of the natural valgus angle in the elbow, supporting the weight of the body on the fully outstretched arm may produce the same medial stretching and lateral compressive forces. In addition, repetitive hyperextension or repetitive traction injuries may occur.

Treatment of Overuse Injuries

One must first recognize that an injury exists. This is not as straightforward as it sounds, for it is often difficult to convince the eager athlete or coach that a problem exists just because the child has some pain after each activity. No obvious deformity or immediate disability may be present, yet if the injury continues, significant long-term disability may result. Proper treatment requires an accurate anatomic diagnosis of the injury and an assessment of the individual's sport activity. In pitching injuries in which no anatomic change has occurred but symptoms persist, an experienced pitching coach can usually alter pitching style to take emphasis away from the side-arm throw, or away from "opening up too fast," and thus often relieve the symptoms of a young pitcher. Weight training, strengthening the forearm flexors and shoulder rotators, as well as flexibility training emphasizing a range of external rotation at the shoulder, can help relieve symptoms about the elbow. However, if symptoms persist, the danger of future damage far outweighs the advantages of continuing to compete in that particular activity. Much progress has been made in restricting the number of innings that may be pitched by Little League participants and restricting practice pitching. Often, however, the eager athlete will continue to practice outside the confines of the league or may even join a second league. Although proper warm-up and gradual assumption of activity will relieve some stress from the elbow, "throwing through" the discomfort will only cause further damage. Surgical excision of loose bodies, drilling of areas of osteonecrosis, debridement of chronic ligamentitis, or other procedures may provide relief but cannot be counted upon to restore normal function. Antiinflammatory drugs or steroid injections probably have no place in treating elbow symptoms in this age group. Early recognition of symptoms, analysis, and alteration or restriction of activities remain the cornerstone of treatment.

Lateral Epicondylitis

This condition is a frequent result of racquet sports in which repetitive action of the forearm and wrist extensors results in a chronic strain of their origin from lateral humeral epicondyli. This is one of the causes of "tennis elbow" in the adult and, because of either increased flexibility or better over-all conditioning, is encountered rarely in the youthful racquet player.

SHOULDER INJURIES

ANATOMY

The complex anatomy of the shoulder includes a shallow ball and socket joint that permits a wide arc of rotation and circumduction. This wide arc of motion makes the sholder inherently less stable and more prone to dislocation than other ball and socket joints such as the hip. Figure 4-16 shows the radiologic anatomy of a growing shoulder, which at times can be confusing. Figure 4-17 shows major anatomic structures including the rotator cuff that provides abduction, and internal and external rotation. Its passage beneath the coracoacromial ligament and its position between the humeral head and overlying acromion make it prone to injury.

EXAMINATION

Examination of the shoulder should include range of motion as compared with the other shoulder and a search for localized tenderness.

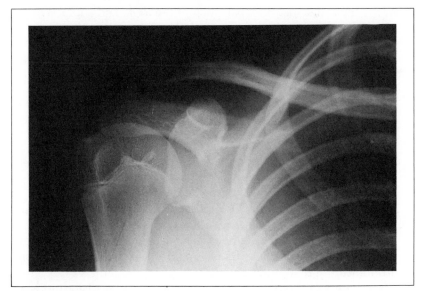

Figure 4-16. Radiologic anatomy of growing shoulder.

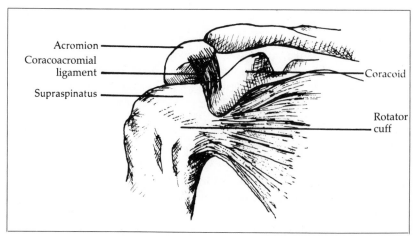

Figure 4-17. Basic anatomy of the shoulder.

Knowledge of the major muscle groups around the shoulder greatly facilitates an accurate examination. Pain on passive motion only suggests an abnormality of the joint or capsular structures, whereas pain on resisted active motion suggests an abnormality of the muscle or tendon responsible for that function. Pain in the shoulder in the absence of local tenderness or positive physical findings suggests referred pain. Common causes of referred pain in the shoulder include lesions of the upper chest or brachial plexus, brachial plexus compression as in thoracic outlet syndrome, nerve root irritation, and referred pain from the cervical spine. Brief palpation of the axilla and supraclavicular area and range of motion of the cervical spine are suggested.

DISLOCATIONS AND SUBLUXATIONS

Dislocations and subluxations of the glenohumeral joint are probably the most common sports-related injury encountered by the team physician. A fall on the abducted or extended arm may produce an anterior and inferior dislocation. Posterior dislocation does also occur. The dislocation is permitted either by extremely lax joint capsules or by tearing a previously taut joint capsule. First-time dislocations are accompanied by much pain and swelling and the appearance of a hollow on the lateral aspect of the shoulder.

Manipulative reduction of the shoulder dislocation should always be preceded by an x-ray and a neurovascular examination. The inferior dislocation may compromise the axillary nerve and give hypoesthesia over the area of the deltoid. Also a humeral neck fracture may occur, contraindicating manipulation without anesthesia and x-ray.

After manipulative reduction most acute shoulder dislocations are immobilized for approximately six weeks followed by a rehabilitation

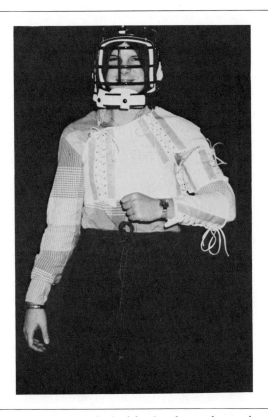

Figure 4-18. Harness restraint to limit abduction, lessen chance of recurrent dislocation.

program. If the shoulder capsule fails to heal completely, if the glenoid labrum has been torn away from the edge of the glenoid, or if the person has inherent capsular laxity, recurrent dislocations may occur. Frequently the athlete is able to reduce these himself. Only if the athlete has had many recurrent dislocations, has no neurovascular involvement, and has had a previous x-ray, is it recommended that dislocations be reduced at the playing field.

Recurrent glenohumeral dislocations can be treated sometimes by muscle strengthening alone but frequently require surgical intervention. For the athlete who wishes to continue to participate without operation or wishes to delay operation, harness type devices (Figure 4-18) limiting shoulder abduction and extension are available.

Recurrent glenohumeral subluxation (partial dislocation without spontaneous relocation) may occur in a variety of sports with or without an antecedent dislocation. Symptoms include giving way, pain on forward elevation or abduction, and feeling the shoulder "go limp." They may be associated with radiating dysesthesias in the arm from brachial plexus compression. Treatment of chronic subluxation includes an attempt to strengthen the shoulder girdle but may often require surgical intervention.

ACROMIOCLAVICULAR JOINT INJURIES

These injuries are common and occur usually with a fall on the point of the shoulder. Extreme lateral flexion of the neck may occur at the same time with an associated brachial plexus injury. The acromioclavicular joint may appear swollen and the distal end of the clavicle may appear subluxated superiorly or posteriorly depending on the grade of subluxation. Plain x-rays that will be normal in a Grade I subluxation will show superior and posterior subluxation of the distal acromion when weights are added to both arms to accentuate the Grade II dislocation and show complete superior and posterior displacement of the clavicle when a Grade III or total separation is present.

The treatment of Grade I sprains of the acromioclavicular joint (no displacement) is purely symptomatic, consisting of sling and appropriate rest until symptoms permit return to activity (about one week or less). The symptoms associated with Grade II sprains (partial displacement) may last longer and some physicians feel these should be treated with an extensive system of strapping. Others treat them symptomatically. Treatment of Grade III sprains (complete displacement) of the acromioclavicular joint is controversial. This author treats almost all Grade III dislocations symptomatically, resorting to operation only in those that are chronically symptomatic. On the other hand, many surgeons prefer acute surgical treatment of the dislocated acromioclavicular joint. Others use a system of strapping. All three grades of sprain may be associated with late acromioclavicular joint symptoms. All of these injuries should be fully rehabilitated before return to activity.

In the young child dislocations of the acromioclavicular joint are uncommon and the same injurious force may cause a fracture of the distal end of the clavicle. Traditional clavicle fracture treatment such as figure-of-eight bandages will tend to distract this fracture farther and a system of strapping as for joint separation should be used.

FRACTURES

Clavicle Fractures

These are extremely common in all types of youth sports. Diaphyseal fractures in the mid-portion of the clavicle vary in the time required to heal from a few weeks in a young child with a displaced fracture to as much as eight weeks in a minimally displaced mid-diaphyseal fracture. These must be treated individually and radiographic union and clinical union demonstrated before a return to violent activity. Returning the child to activity when symptoms permit, but before radiographic union, puts him at risk for development of delayed union. However, the child involved in a pure running sport obviously may return earlier.

Injuries to the Medial Clavicle and Sternoclavicular Joint

Forward propulsion of the shoulder or a lateral blow on the shoulder may dislocate the sternoclavicular joint or fracture the medial end of the clavicle. In a growing child the medial end of the clavicle contains a growing epiphysis and fractures occur here commonly, mimicking dislocations. Rarely, the medial end of the clavicle is dislocated posteriorly into the chest and this may be a life-threatening situation because of compromise of the great vessels or pneumothorax. The more common anterior dislocation of the medial end of the clavicle is a perplexing situation for which the surgical treatment is difficult and the nonsurgical generally unsatisfactory. These injuries should be referred.

Overuse Injuries

Throwing Injuries

Shoulder injuries in throwing sports are almost as common as elbow injuries. Most throwing acts necessitate full abduction, extension, and external rotation of the shoulder. In this position the anterior capsular structures and subscapularis muscle tendon are placed under stress and may become inflamed with repetitive use.

On the "follow through" portion of throwing, the posterior capsule or teres minor may become stretched or there may be impingement of the humerus on the anterior glenoid neck. A chronic rotator cuff impingement syndrome may result from repetitive circumduction. In general, a greater arc of motion will make these injuries less likely and greater strength of the muscles of the shoulder girdle will make them less likely. Analysis of these overuse injuries requires a thorough knowledge of the shoulder anatomy and the sport involved. Often the most help comes from an experienced throwing coach who can alter throwing style once the anatomic origin of the problem is understood.

Rotator Cuff Injuries and Chronic Impingement Syndrome

The rotator cuff, a conjoined unit of tendon and capsule from the infraspinatus, supraspinatus, and subscapularis muscles, envelops the humeral head and provides most of the forces of rotation and abduction (see Figure 4-17). This structure must pass beneath the coracoacromial ligament and between the humeral head and acromion. In this vulnerable position it may be chronically pinched or irritated. The increased inflammation of the tendon and swelling diminish the clearance available for it in motion and a cycle of inflammation and increased impingement may occur. This is generally felt to be the cause of most adult shoulder "tendinitis" or "bursitis" and rarely occurs in the young athlete unless a repetitive upper extremity sport involving throwing or abduction or chronic use of the shoulder in an abducted or extended position is encountered. This is a common injury in swimmers. Rarely, the young athlete with a single traumatic event may avulse the insertion of the rotator cuff or actually tear the rotator cuff, resulting in shoulder swelling and inability to abduct the arm. Persistent limitation of active abduction should make one suspicious of a rotator cuff tear. This may be diagnosed by arthrogram and, although a repair may be accomplished at a later time, it is best done acutely. Treatment of rotator cuff impingement syndromes is frustrating because of the inherent anatomic limitations imposed by the acromion and coracoacromial ligament. Standard treatments include antiimflammatories, rest, shoulder girdle strengthening to try to depress the humeral head and allow more clearance for the rotator cuff, alteration in sport technique, and finally surgery. Little is documented about the success of surgical treatment of this injury in athletes.

Shoulder problems in swimming may be the limiting factor in an athlete's career. The repetitive abduction and the circumduction of movements involved in the breast stroke and especially in the butterfly stroke frequently give rise to chronic impingement syndrome. Once this syndrome is recognized some help may be obtained by altering swimming style, but usually the athlete's participation in a given event will have to be restricted. Many swimmers "save" their shoulders for competition and minimize training in the strokes that cause symptoms. Unlike chronic elbow problems from throwing, chronic shoulder symptoms in the competitive swimmer seem to subside when activity is stopped and rarely leave residual disability. Occasionally a stress fracture of the upper humerus may mimic chronic impingement syndrome.

Brachial Plexus Injuries

The brachial plexus is of a relatively fixed length and when the neck is laterally flexed or rotated and the shoulder depressed, it is stretched. This occurs commonly on a fall to the side, particularly when a helmet helps force the head laterally. The brachial plexus may be stretched transiently or seriously damaged.

Burners

These injuries occur commonly in football when the head and shoulder are used in tackling. A brief electric or shooting discomfort is felt in the area of the trapezius, shoulder, or upper arm for at most a few seconds. This represents a transient stretch to the brachial plexus. Use of a "horse collar" or other supportive device to the neck such as straps from the shoulder pads to the helmet to limit lateral flexion may control symptoms. Preseason neck strengthening exercises may prevent these symptoms. If burners become persistent in spite of these measures, a search for a cervical spine injury should be made, including neurological examination, x-ray, and probably flexion extension films. Burners should be distinguished from cervical radiculitis or signs of cervical spine injury. Symptoms lasting more than a few seconds, simultaneous bilateral symptoms, associated weakness, and radiation to the arm or hand are adequate reasons to restrict participation pending investigation of the cervical spine.

Occasionally chronic neuropathies around the shoulder of the axillary nerve, supraclavicular nerve, or other branches of the brachial plexus may occur in response to repeated trauma. Muscle wasting about the shoulder with symptoms of weakness should suggest this possibility and lead to referral.

ADDITIONAL READING

EXAMINATION AND EVALUATION OF THE INJURED HAND

Edmunson, A. (Ed.) *Campbell's Operative Orthopaedics* (6th ed.). St. Louis: Mosby, 1980.

Hoppenfeld, S. *Physical Examination of the Spine and Extremities.* New York: Appleton-Century-Crofts, 1976.

Kalenak, A., et. al. Athletic injuries of the hand. *Am. Fam. Physician* 14: 136, 1976.

Milford, L. The Hand. In A. Edmunson (Ed.), *Campbell's Operative Orthopaedics* (6th ed.). St. Louis: Mosby, 1980.

SPLINTING HAND INJURIES

MacCollum, M. S. Protecting upper extremity injuries in sports. *Physiol. Sports Med.* 8:59, 1980.

ELBOW INJURIES

Brown, R., et. al. Osteochondritis of the capitellum. *J. Sports Med.* 2:27, 1974.

Dehaven, K. E. Elbow problems in the adolescent athlete. *Cleveland Clin. Q.* 42:297, 1975.

DeHaven, K. E., and Everts, C. M. Throwing injuries of the elbow in athletes. *Orthop, Clin. North Am.* 4:801, 1973.

Gugenheim, J. J., et. al. Little League survey: The Houston study. *Am. J. Sports Med.* 4:189, 1976.

Larson, R. L., et al. Little League survey: The Eugene study. *Am. J. Sports Med.* 4:201, 1976.

SHOULDER INJURIES

Albright, J. A., et al. Clinical study of baseball pitchers: Correlation of injury to the throwing arm with method of delivery. *Am. J. Sports Med.* 6:15, 1978.

Dominguez, R. H. Shoulder pain in swimmers. *Physiol. Sports Med.* 8:37, 1980.

Jackson, D. W. Chronic rotator cuff impingement in the throwing athlete. *Am. J. Sports Med.* 4:231, 1976.

Leach, R. E., O'Connor, P., and Jones, R. Acromionectomy for tendinitis of the shoulder in athletes. *Physiol. Sports Med.* 7:96, 1979.

Norwood, L. A., et al. Anterior shoulder pain in baseball pitchers. *Am. J. Sports Med.* 6:103, 1978.

5. Lower Limb Injuries in Childhood and Adolescence

Philip J. Mayer

Growth is the quality that differentiates preadolescents and adolescents from adults. Kennedy [20] defines "adolescence" as the years between 12 and 18. During preadolescence, the growth plates are all open and growing rapidly. During adolescence, epiphyseal plates slowly begin to close and various supporting structures about the joints of the lower extremity are first subjected to overuse syndromes and the risks of contact sports. There is now some evidence to show that the preadolescent athlete, even when engaged in organized football, is less at risk for injury than the high-school or college-level player [26]. Roser and Clawson [35] found a 2.3 percent rate of injury among 2,097 participants in the Seattle Junior Football League. Godshall [15] found only two major injuries (fractures of the leg) and a few minor fractures (wrist, fingers, and foot) when he reviewed the records of the Pop Warner football program in Pennsylvania in which 1,700 boys had participated during a 12-year period. Furthermore, Pop Warner officials have not reported a mortality in their first 43 years of existence during which more than 1 million children registered for football programs.

There is now some new data that indicate the incidence of injuries in grade-school athletes is both significant and on the increase. As the child grows into adolescence, the injury rate has been shown to increase. The *Neiss Report* [29] recording the following adolescent injuries from a variety of activities between May 1976 and May 1977 suggests the extent of the problem.

Baseball	362,651
Basketball	348,389
Bicycling	450,331
Football	381,844
Snow skiing	80,263
Swings, slides, seesaws, and climbing apparatus	137,355

In 1955, O'Donoghue [30] noted that 55 percent of his patients with surgically treated knees were less than 20 years of age, but that only one patient was less than 15 years of age. Recent data have pointed to an increase in lower limb injuries in this age group over the past 20 years. Garrick and Requa [14] reviewed injury patterns in 3, 534 child and adolescent skiers. They found an injury rate of 9.1 per 1,000 skier days. Injury rates increased steadily with increasing age up to 13 years of age, leveled off from 13 to 15 years, and then decreased slightly through age 17.

Sprains were the most common type of injury seen, accounting for 51 percent of all injuries. Contusions were the next most common (17.3%), followed by fractures (11.1%). Students less than 10 years had the lowest incidence of injury. There was no evidence from their study that the open growth plate leads to a higher incidence of epiphyseal injury. Sprains most frequently involved the knee and the ankle.

Nearly two-thirds of the fractures involved the leg and the ankle. The female was more prone to injury than the male. Tapper [40] analyzed 4,227 ski injuries that occurred from 1972 to 1976 at Sun Valley, Idaho, and compared his findings with previous studies dating back to 1939. He found that improvements in safety bindings and boot manufacture have not benefitted children, as reflected in the fact that there has been a steady increase in the percentage of tibial shaft fractures in children. When looking at ski injuries with respect to age, it was found that 32 percent of spiral fractures of the tibia occurred in children age 10 and under. Nilsson and Roaas [29], in reviewing soccer injuries in adolescents, concluded that adolescents playing soccer suffered fewer and less severe injuries than adults. Contusions were the most frequent type of injury and the number of fractures was low. In all regions except the ankle, the number of contusions exceeded the number of sprains. They concluded that adolescents may be protected by having higher elasticity in their skeletal systems and that the force moments generated at impact would be less than in the adult.

Severe injury to the knee in pediatric patients more commonly produces fractures and epiphyseal injuries than ligament injuries, presumably because the resiliency and strength of the ligaments are greater than those of the physis and bone. However, recent reports of knee ligament injuries in children have emphasized the point that ligament injury must be considered in the differential diagnosis of the child suffering from knee trauma [5,23,37].

Because the child is still growing, damage to the growing bones and joints of the lower extremities is the chief danger in childhood injuries. Although children may sustain a typical adult injury, including sprains, strains, contusions, and fractures, they are also susceptible to growth plate injuries, injuries to the epiphysis or end of the bone, avulsions of major musculotendon insertions from bone, and certain overuse injuries to the bones, cartilage, and musculotendon structures of the limbs. Injuries to each anatomic region of the lower extremity will now be discussed.

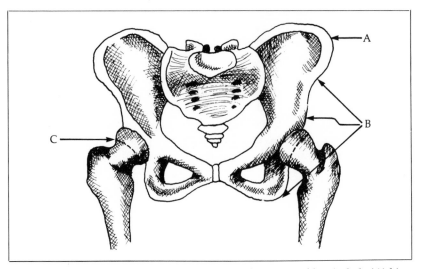

Figure 5-1. Injuries about the hips and pelvis in the young athlete include (A) hip pointers, (B) apophyseal avulsions, and (C) slipped capital femoral epiphysis.

HIP INJURIES

Musculotendon avulsions and contusions are the most common injuries of the hip and pelvis in the young athlete (Figure 5-1).

HIP POINTER (BRUISE OF THE PELVIC CREST)

In all collision sports, appropriate protective padding should be worn over the sides and crests of the pelvis. If protective padding is inadequate, bruises of the upper edge of the pelvis (iliac crest) can occur. This injury is frequently referred to as a "hip pointer." Such bruises or contusions may be excessively painful. Because the abdominal muscles as well as the hip abductor and flexor muscles insert on the iliac crest, motion of these muscles will aggravate the pain. Treatment usually consists of ice compresses and restriction of activity until symptoms subside. Occasionally, the patient may require crutches for protected ambulation for a few days. Sometimes the patient will develop a post-traumatic periostitis of the iliac crest, and the crest will continue to remain painful and tender. This condition will respond in most instances to an injection of local anesthetic and a steroid preparation. At the time of the injection, it is wise to caution the patient that after two hours, when the local anesthetic wears off, his pain may recur and may become more severe than prior to the injection. He should treat his symptoms with ice applications and aspirin as necessary. The pain will then diminish during the next 24 hours.

It is of importance to determine the exact nature of the injury about the pelvic bones (ilium) since the treatment and the protective equipment, as well as the immediate prognosis, will depend in large part upon which muscles are actually involved. Palpation of a defect usually indicates avulsion of a muscle or group of muscles. If there is complete avulsion, surgical repair should be carried out promptly. However, complete avulsion from the iliac crest rarely occurs. Most of these injuries resolve with the simple measures noted above. If the athlete is permitted to return to activity prior to complete healing of his lesion, these injuries may tend to recur. Fracture of the wing of the ilium is not frequent but must be considered if the patient has sustained a direct blow against the pelvic bone. The patient will have severe pain, and muscle spasm will generally prevent deep palpation. Any attempt at function involving the muscles in that area will be painful. Diagnosis can be established by obtaining appropriate x-rays.

Avulsions

Avulsion injuries about the hip are not uncommon. Several large muscle groups insert or originate from about the hip. The iliopsoas tendon, the strongest hip flexor, descends across the superior pubic ramus to insert into the lesser trochanter of the proximal-medial femur. The hip adductor muscles originate from the inferior pubic ramus. Hamstring muscles originate from the posteriorly located ischium and the abductors attach to the greater trochanter. These attachments are called apophyses. An apophysis is a growth area that does not participate in or form port of a joint. These attachments are particularly prone to avulsion injuries during sudden or violent muscle contractions (Figure 5-2). The apophysis may completely avulse or only partially separate. Diagnosis is established clinically by palpating for tenderness and by eliciting pain on the appropriate resisted movements. Avulsion injuries require immediate bed rest, icing of the area, and strong pain medication. As the amount of displacement is generally minimal, satifactory healing can be expected to occur if proper rest and immobilization of the extremity are provided. Surgery is only rarely indicated to restore the muscle to its site of insertion. The more common avulsion injuries are discussed below.

A straddling injury caused by forceful abduction of the thighs may cause damage to the adductor muscles. They may either avulse from their insertion in the ischiopubic rami or tear along their substance. Diagnosis is confirmed by pain on forceful passive abduction of the thigh and on active adduction against resistance. Occasionally, the detachment or rupture may be recognized by a bunching-up of the adductor muscle a short distance away from the pelvis and by a tender-firm mass that is more noticeable on active resisted adduction of the thigh. If this situation is recognized, immediate primary surgical repair is generally indicated.

Overactive contraction of the iliopsoas muscle when the thigh is

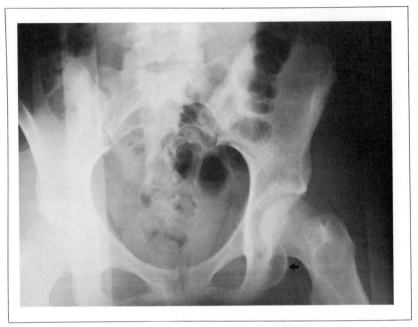

Figure 5-2. Avulsion of the hamstring apophysis from the ischium in a young high jumper. These avulsions can be very painful and disabling, but rarely require surgical repair.

flexed and then forced into extension may result in either a strain of the muscle or an avulsion of its insertion into the lesser trochanter. If the injury is at the lesser trochanter, then tenderness will be below the level of the groin along the upper anteriomedial aspect of the thigh. X-ray confirmation of this diagnosis can usually be made. Even with complete avulsion, surgical repair is rarely indicated as the lesser trochanter reattaches with fibrous union and is usually not painful. Protection should be used, with immobilization in bed with the thigh flexed and externally rotated, and ice compresses should be applied in the early stages. This problem usually requires several weeks for symptoms to subside. Early return to activities may cause a recurrence as any effort to run or jump will cause excessive strain on this tendon. It must be emphasized that the iliopsoas is an important flexor of the thigh and that complete recovery is necessary before unrestricted function can be permitted.

SLIPPED CAPITAL FEMORAL EPIPHYSIS

Although injuries to the articular cartilage of the femoral head or the acetabulum are relatively rare, since the hip is a deep joint well protected by soft tissue, occasionally minimal trauma can precipitate the slipping of the femoral shaft with respect to the femoral head across the epiphyseal growth plate. The condition is encountered most frequently in adolescence (boys 13–16 years; girls, 11–14 years). It rarely occurs in girls following menarche. Characteristically, the condition tends to occur in individuals of two body types: more commonly in those who are large, obese, and sexually immature, and less often in those who are tall and thin. The presenting complaint is usually pain in the region of the groin referred to the anteromedial aspect of the thigh and knee. Knee pain may be the only presenting complaint. The patient has a painful limp and holds the lower extremity in an externally rotated position. Internal rotation, abduction, and flexion of the affected hip are usually limited. X-ray confirmation is necessary to establish the diagnosis. Treatment for the condition is surgical.

THIGH

Anatomically, the thigh consists of a single bone, the femur, completely surrounded by very heavy muscles. Anterior is the quadriceps muscle mass. Medial is the adductor muscle mass. Posterior are the hamstring muscles. The hamstring muscles are particularly susceptible to strain-type injuries. These strain injuries may involve either tears of the muscle or avulsion of the origin into the ischium. The large anterior quadriceps muscle, on the other hand, is frequently injured by contusion in contact sports, such as football, since the thigh often receives the brunt of the collision force between participants. Contusion results in a painful limp caused by swelling, and accumulation of blood within the muscle, and restricted hip and knee ranges of motion. The symptoms of muscle contusion are less well localized than those of contusions in the more superficial subcutaneous tissue. The patient may not be disabled at the time of the blow, but will gradually develop aching, soreness, and swelling within the muscle. Often, there develops a sympathetic effusion in the knee joint. Range of motion will be limited due to the pain caused by tension on the swollen muscle fibers.

Myositis Ossificans

An unfortunate sequela of thigh contusion may be the development of myositis ossificans, which is the formation of heterotopic bone within the muscle substance. The etiology of myositis ossificans is unknown. It is probably related to the presence of blood and concomitant inflammatory reaction within the muscle. Prompt recognition of thigh contusions and hematoma formation and appropriate initial treatment may avert the development of myositis ossificans.

Treatment for thigh contusions consists of initial ice compresses and immobilization. I prefer to apply a compressive dressing that is a modification of a Robert Jones splint. This consists of inner layers of either cotton or cast padding with plaster splints placed medially and laterally, over which a gentle compressive gauze wrap is placed followed by elastic bandages. This dressing extends from the ankle to the groin, and a separate plastic bandage is wrapped gently about the foot to prevent swelling of the distal extremity. Some prefer to infiltrate muscle hematomas with hyaluronidase, which may hasten resorption of the hematoma [31,33]. The compressive dressing should be continued as long as the thigh remains tense and swollen. Initially, the patient may have to be put at bed rest with the leg elevated, prior to being ambulated with crutches. As the swelling begins to subside the patient may begin gradual active range-of-motion exercises within the limits of pain. O'Donoghue emphasized that there is no place for massage in the early treatment of contusion of the muscle. Such kneading of the injured muscle merely serves to increase the damage.

In a small percentage of patients, healing of the injured quadriceps muscle fails to occur within the usual 10–14 days. Swelling persists and motion of the knee, and occasionally of the hip, gradually becomes more limited. A mass can often be palpated at about three weeks following the injury, and x-rays will often show evidence of new bone formation within the muscle. It is common for myositis ossificans to develop over a period of several weeks and to take as long as six months to resolve. The size of the bone mass may vary from a few millimeters to one that is quite large and incapacitating. Once myositis ossificans has developed, the treatment must be one of gradual re-habilitation exercises with active range-of-motion exercises using pain as a guideline. At no time should the patient be subjected to forceful manipulation of the involved extremity as this may lead to more bleeding and a worsening of the condition. Likewise, early surgical intervention has been shown to be followed by recurrence of the bony mass. On rare occasions, the bony mass may mature and fail to resolve. If it is large and interferes with the function of the muscle, and if it has been established that the process has reached a stage of maturity, then one may consider surgical excision. It is important to be aware of the entity myositis ossificans because in its early stage its x-ray appearance may mimic that of an osteogenic sarcoma. The clinical history is extremely important in the differential diagnosis as it is quite difficult to distinguish by pathological examination between the early growing bone of a myositis ossificans and the early osteogenesis of a sarcoma of the bone.

THE INJURED KNEE

Knee injuries in children are a particularly important subject. Gross-man and Nicholas [17] have pointed out that common afflictions of the knee due to athletic injury are becoming a matter of serious concern to physicians. In sports, the knee provides the needed balance for support, agility, and precise activity, and it is frequently at risk be-

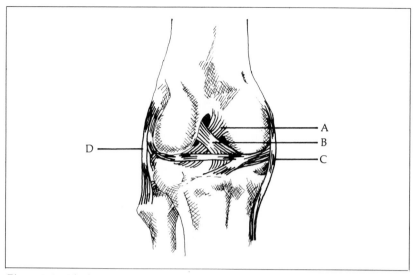

Figure 5-3. The knee and its ligaments, seen from behind the knee. The major ligaments include (A) the anterior cruciate, (B) the posterior cruciate, (C) the medial collateral, and (D) the lateral collateral.

cause of its relatively exposed position. Additionally, the knee must transmit large forces for both acceleration and deceleration and for changes of direction during the performance of many sports activities. As noted above, although knee ligament injuries in children have been shown to be rare, they do occur, and they are being recognized with increasing frequency (Figure 5-3). In addition to fractures and ligamentous injuries, the growing knee is at risk to develop a variety of problems not seen in the adult. Kennedy has recently published a book entitled *The Injured Adolescent Knee* [20] that deals specifically with problems encountered in the growing knee and this source is recommended for further reading.

Common disorders of the knee have been categorized according to four age groups: youth (5–17 years), prime (17–35 years), adult (35–55 years), and senior age group (above 55 years) [16]. The most common disorders found in youth are developmental problems such as osteochondritis dissecans, discoid menisci, and Osgood–Schlatter's disease. Other disorders frequent in youth are chondromalacia patella, perhaps better thought of as patellofemoral pain syndrome, meniscal injuries, capsular tears, and epiphyseal fractures. Common disorders in the prime age group are ligamentous injury, chondromalacia and patellar pain, meniscal injury, patella tendinitis, osteochondritis dissecans and osteochondral fractures, knee dislocations, fractures, and osteoarthritis secondary to degenerative changes. Developmental problems are said to be the primary reason that people between 5 and 17 years of age seek orthopedic consultation.

Treatment of the Injured Knee

The history is important and one must determine as accurately as possible the mechanism of injury, the presence and nature of swelling, pain, and locking, as well as any history of having heard a "pop" or "snap" at the time of injury. It is important to know if this is the first injury or if there has been any knee problem in the past or a past history of trauma.

By knowing the mechanism of injury, it is sometimes possible to predict the pathology of injury. One should try to determine whether the knee was flexed or extended, whether the tibia was rotated internally or externally, and whether the knee was weight-bearing or non-weight-bearing.

A weight-bearing knee may well injure a meniscus, whereas ligamentous injuries would be more common in the unweighted knee. A valgus stress with the knee in flexion and the tibia externally rotated, as might occur in a clipping injury in football, would jeopardize the medial collateral ligamentous structures, the anterior cruciate ligament, and the medial meniscus. Although varus injuries are unusual, they would implicate the lateral collateral ligament.

A hyperextension injury, especially with a history of hearing a "pop" in the knee followed by acute onset of swelling, would make one think of an anterior cruciate ligament tear. Extreme hyperextension, as might occur during a football tackle, could avulse the posterior cruciate ligament as well as tear the posterior joint capsule. A rotational component to the injury usually means that the damage sustained will be more severe, and one should think of meniscal damage and patella dislocation in addition to ligament tears.

The history of acute swelling in an injured knee most frequently means hemarthrosis, and Eriksson [18, 19] has stated that the most common reason for acute hemarthrosis is injury to the anterior cruciate ligament. A painful, tense effusion means that the joint capsule is intact, whereas in a more severe injury with capsular damage, the joint will decompress itself into the soft tissue. Pain may not develop until 12–24 hours after the injury in grade I to grade II ligament sprains and may take one to two weeks to resolve. On the other hand, complete ligament tears (grade III), due to the decompressive effect of the capsular tear, may be quite painless.

Locking may be classified as true or mechanical locking and pseudo-locking. True locking, as seen with a torn meniscus, loose body in the joint, or blocking of motion by the remnant of the torn cruciate ligament, is generally painless. On the other hand, pseudo-locking associated with ligament tears and patellofemoral pain symptoms is associated with effusion, pain, and muscle spasms.

The history of a "pop" or "snap" in the knee at the time of injury has been said by Marshall [22] to indicate anterior cruciate ligament rupture in greater than 90 percent of patients giving this history. On the other hand, Marshall notes that 65 percent of people with anterior cruciate ligament injury did not give a history of a "pop." A painless, unpredictable "giving-way" is often suggestive of an anterior cruciate ligament–insufficient knee with significant instability. On the other hand, a "collapsing knee" associated with pain prior to collapsing may indicate patellofemoral problems, muscular weakness, or mechanical locking.

History of pain in the posterior aspect of the joint experienced on deep squatting may be associated with a torn meniscus. The presence of an intermittently palpable firm bulge, which may often have to be pushed back into place, may indicate the presence of loose bodies ("joint mice").

Finally, it must be emphasized that the managing medical personnel must maintain a high index of suspicion when dealing with the acutely injured knee. No longer must we be satisfied with the initial diagnosis of "internal derangement of the knee" and a management plan that consists of placing the acutely injured knee in a cylinder cast for two weeks for the purpose of reassessing it at the end of that time. We know now that such treatment may result in the physician missing the golden period of time during the first few days after injury during which ligament repair rather than reconstruction can be performed. In all instances, early repair of acutely damaged structures is more desirable than having to do delayed reconstructive procedures.

PHYSICAL EXAMINATION

To accurately evaluate the acutely injured knee, a detailed history and carefully organized physical examination must be performed. It is essential to keep in mind the general classification of ligament sprains that divides them into three grades: mild, moderate, and severe [18, 20]. A grade I, or mild, sprain is a microscopic tearing of the ligament in which there is local tenderness, minimal swelling, no instability, and little disability. A grade II, or moderate, sprain indicates a loss of the integrity of the ligament due to microscopic and gross disrupture of the ligamentous fibers. There will be local tenderness, swelling, slight to moderate instability, and moderate disability. Physical examination will reveal definite laxity but a firm end-point should be felt. A grade III, or severe, sprain is a complete loss of anatomical integrity of the ligament, with marked instability, severe disability, tenderness, swelling, hemorrhage, and an absent or "mushy" endpoint on examination.

The injured knee must be evaluated for swelling, deformity, tender areas, range of motion, and instability. Observation may reveal abrasions, gross evidence of swelling, or loss of the visible joint contours particularly in the suprapatellar region. Palpation will reveal evidence of an effusion. To test for an effusion, one should compress the suprapatellar pouch and try to ballott the patella by pressing it up and down against the femur. Small effusions can be identified by causing a fluid wave to shift from side to side underneath the patella. Palpation should be done over the medial collateral ligamentous structures at the femoral insertion of the superficial medial collateral ligament, the deep meniscofemoral ligament just above the joint line, the mensicus peripheral margin at the joint line, the deep meniscotibial ligament below the joint line, and the insertion of the superficial medial collateral ligament three finger breadths below the joint line on the medial aspect of the tibial metaphysis. Palpation should also identify areas of tenderness, particularly at the level of the epiphyseal growth plates of both the femur and the tibia. By placing the knee in a figure-of-four position, it is possible to palpate the tense lateral collateral ligament as it inserts on the fibular head. Palpation must be done along both sides of the patella. This may elicit medial retinacular tenderness or a feeling of a void in that area should a tear have occurred with a dislocated patella. Palpation of the undersurface of the patella facets may elicit tenderness in a patient with chondromalacia patella or patellofemoral pain syndrome. With the knee in 5 to 10 degrees of flexion, force can be applied to the medial border of the patella, thus displacing it laterally. Normally, there will be no response from the patient; however, in someone with a subluxing patella, as the patella tends to ride laterally, the patient can become quite apprehensive and either tense his quadriceps muscle or actually grasp the examiner's hand. This test is appropriately known as the "apprehension test."

In order to fully evaluate an injured knee, it is necessary to have a relaxed, cooperative patient. Unfortunately, this period of time is rather brief, and shortly after the injury, with the onset of pain, swelling, and spasm, examination will prove to be difficult. It may be necessary to aspirate a tense hematoma for diagnostic purposes while instilling 5–10 ml 1% Xylocaine into the joint as a local anesthetic. Range of motion should be tested, but this may be difficult in the acutely injured knee. For proper diagnosis and treatment, simple stability tests must be performed. These are done in both the anterior and posterior, and the medial-lateral, planes. A valgus stress should be applied to the knee in full extension, which tests for the integrity of the posteromedial joint capsule and the posterior cruciate ligament, and then in 30 degrees of flexion, which tests more specifically the integrity of the medial collateral ligamentous complex. Likewise, a varus stress test should be done with the knee in extension and in 30 degrees of flexion. Tests for anterior-posterior instability are done with the patient lying down, the knee flexed to 90 degrees and the foot resting firmly on the table. The examiner should actually sit on the dorsum of the patient's foot to stabilize the extremity. With the foot pointing straight ahead, an anterior drawer sign and posterior drawer sign may be elicited. These reflect the integrity of the anterior cruciate and posterior cruciate ligaments, respectively. With the foot externally rotated, the posteromedial joint capsule and structures are tightened, and a positive drawer test indicates disruption to this area as well as a probable tear of the anterior cruciate ligament. A positive drawer test done with the foot internally rotated indicates the presence of an anterolateral rotatory instability, which is often associated with insufficiency of the anterior cruciate ligament and the posterior lateral capsule. Torg [41] has suggested that the anterior drawer sign be done with the knee in extension (Lachman's test), because laboratory studies have shown with the anterior cruciate ligament torn, anterior tibial displacement is greatest in the extended knee. Torg has emphasized that the character of the end-point for interpretation must be "mushy" as opposed to hard or firm. However, in practice with a large extremity, it is difficult to perform Lachman's test.

Recently, the pivot shift (lateral pivot shift, jerk test) has been popularized by MacIntosh and Galloway [12, 13]. A positive lateral pivot shift demonstrates the presence of anterolateral rotatory instability and represents the subluxation of the lateral tibial plateau anteriorly on the femoral condyle. The test is done by having the patient lie in a supine position and grasping the foot with one hand while placing the other hand posterior to the proximal fibula. The tibia is then internally rotated and valgus stress is applied to the knee. The knee is flexed and extended and an actual jerk or clunk may be felt as subluxation occurs in 5 to 10 degrees of flexion. With further flexion, the tibia relocates as a similar jerk is felt. In order to perform this test, it is absolutely necessary that the patient be fully relaxed. I frequently perform this test prior to the rest of the knee examination because once the patient becomes sensitized to any painful stimuli, he or she is unlikely to relax enough to elicit a positive lateral pivot shift.

COMMON KNEE INJURIES

OSTEOCHONDRITIS DISSECANS

Osteochondritis dissecans is a lesion that occurs most often on the articular surface of the femoral condyles, especially on the lateral aspect of the medial femoral condyle. On x-ray, it is seen as a radiolucent line demarcating a small area of subchondral bone on the medial side of the interchondylar notch, and is best seen on the tunnel view (Figure 5-4). It most often occurs in the adolescent age group but has been reported in children as young as 4 years old [17, 34]. The etiology has been attributed by various authors to trauma, ischemia, epiphyseal developmental abnormalities, and hereditary factors. The patient usually presents with a history of intermittent nonspecific knee pain usually related to some form of exercise. Activities that cause repetitive flexion-extension movements of the knees such as running or bicycle

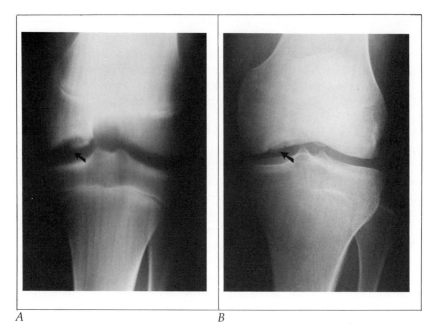

Figure 5-4. Osteochondritis dissecans, as seen on tomograms of an adolescent knee (A), or as a persistent defect and source of pain in the adult (B).

riding have been reported to cause slight swelling and soreness. The child may complain of stiffness, swelling, clicking, and locking of the knee. There may be an associated limp. Physical examination may localize a point of tenderness over the lesion by flexing the knees to 90 degrees and palpating the anterior surface of the femoral condyle. Quadriceps muscle atrophy is common. The lesion may be bilateral in 25 to 30 percent of the juvenile group [16]. Treatment depends on the age of the patient, the location and extent of the fragment, and the clinical presentation of the patient. The prognosis for spontaneous healing of the nondetached lesion in children is excellent. Children may heal without immobilization, but if symptoms persist, then cylinder cast immobilization with the knee flexed to approximately 30 degrees may be necessary for a period of several weeks. Intermittent periods of discomfort may be relieved by home use of Buck's traction or a removable knee splint. The patient should be started on isometric quadriceps strengthening exercises as soon as possible and these should be continued throughout his course of treatment. Healing usually takes place in 6 to 12 months. Surgery is indicated if the fragment becomes detached and loose within the joint. Depending on the size of the fragment, it may either be removed with the bed being drilled, or be reattached with small pins.

Osgood–Schlatter's disease

Osgood–Schlatter's disease is one of the most frequent causes of knee pain in young athletes [27]. It is generally thought to be an apophysitis or inflammation of the patella tubercle at the site of insertion of the quadriceps muscle through the patella into the tibia. It appears frequently in the young male adolescent who is quite active. It is characterized by pain over the tibial tubercle area with swelling against resistance, whereas the patient can usually maintain a strong painless quadriceps isometric contraction in the extended position. Symptoms are aggravated by activities that require repetitive quadriceps contractions such as running or jumping. X-ray examination may reveal swelling and fragmentation of the tibial tubercle on the lateral view. Treatment is directed at controlling the symptoms by the use of rest and antiinflammatory medications such as aspirin 10 gr 4 times a day. Once the symptoms have been controlled, the patient is started on quadriceps isometric and hamstring isotonic progressive resistive exercises. These are performed once a day doing 3 sets of 10 repetitions with each exercise. By doing quadriceps isometric exercises with the knee extended, the extension force is diffused through the medial and lateral retinacula of the knee and symptoms are not aggravated. Additionally, during the course of treatment, the patient is able to rehabilitate his thigh musculature so that, as the disease runs its course, he is better able to resume activities. Injection of steroids into the area of the patella tendon and tibial tubercle are not to be recommended as degenerative changes may occur in the patella tendon leading to subsequent rupture [17, 18, 19].

Discoid Menisci

The discoid meniscus, although rare, must be considered in the adolescent presenting with a history of "snap" or "click" experienced with the knee between 0 and 30 degrees flexion. The "click" can usually be reproduced by doing a McMurray's circumduction test in which the knee is first flexed and the tibia internally rotated and then extended. As this examination is done, the fingers can often palpate a "click" or "clunk" along the lateral joint line. Arthrograms and arthroscopy will confirm the diagnosis and the treatment is surgical if the symptoms warrant it.

Patellofemoral Pain Syndrome (Chondromalacia Patella)

Pain in the patellofemoral joint frequently causes disabling symptoms in young people, who then seek medical advice. The problem affects male and female athletes as well as the more classically described knock-kneed, obese female. The patella may be thought as "the great masquerader" [22] in that it is quite easy to confuse patellofemoral pain with symptoms of meniscal or ligamentous injuries unless a carefully detailed history is taken. Patellofemoral pain can occur at any age. It is a particularly difficult problem in young people. Since the term *chondromalacia patella* is actually a pathological diagnosis, it is more appropriate to term the initial diagnosis as "patellofemoral pain syndrome," unless there is evidence of gross and/or microscopic degeneration of the patella cartilage.

Although chondromalacia patella has commonly been thought to occur more frequently in females, we have noted a male predominance of 3 to 2 in our population of athletes [7]. One-third of our patients have a history of specific injury. Symptoms were bilateral in one-third and chronic (persisting for more than six months) in two-thirds of the patients interviewed. It is important to ask the patient whether a frank patella dislocation has occurred in the past, and, if so, whether its etiology was traumatic or habitual. For example, did the patient receive a direct blow to the knee or did the knee merely twist to one side? A history of instability (such as giving-way) and subsequent swelling may indicate recurrent subluxation. Some patients (25 percent in our series) complained of grating or crepitus. There may also be a history of catching or "locking" as the knee moves through a range of motion. Although pain is the most common presenting complaint, up to one-fourth of the patients do not cite pain as their chief complaint. These patients may be more affected by stiffness, grating, locking, or painless giving-way due to ligamentous instability. Typically, the pain occurs when the patellofemoral joint is undergoing loading and flexion (e.g., ascending and descending stairs) or prolonged sitting with the knee flexed, as the patellofemoral compression forces are greatly increased with the knee in a flexed position. The patient may also experience pain and/or stiffness when he begins to walk after having sat for a long period of time ("movie" sign). Although the pain can usually be localized to the peripatellar area, it may also be felt anteromedially and anterolaterally, and, occasionally, posteriorly. It may occur either during or after activity.

The physical examination must be done with care and precision. One must look carefully for evidence of patella malalignment. Malalignment is typically seen in the patient with increased femoral anteversion, compensatory external tibial torsion, and pronation of the feet. When the patient stands with feet together, the patellae may be positioned anteriomedially (squinting patellae) if there is increased femoral anteversion and increased quadriceps or Q-angle as measured from the anterior superior iliac spine to the middle of the patella to the tibial tubercle. The Q-angle is abnormal if it exceeds 15 degrees. Such a grouping of deformities is common in the chondromalacia knee.

Retropatellar tenderness can be elicited by direct palpation of the medial and lateral facets as the patella is displaced to one side and then the other with the knee extended and the patient relaxed. Tenderness may also be elicited by palpation along the joint line, which may be suggestive of a meniscal tear. As noted above, apprehension may be elicited as a sign of instability. I also perform the dynamic patella compression test by compressing the superior aspect of the patella between the thumb and index finger as the patient actively tightens the quadriceps in a position of 10 degrees flexion. A positive test results in pain, which occurs in 70 percent of the patients. When the patient sits with his knees flexed at 90 degrees and the patella face up and out, one can make the presumptive diagnosis of patella alta (high-riding patella) that is associated with patellofemoral pain. One should also look for the presence of an effusion and thigh-girth atrophy measuring 15 cm above the inferior pole of the patella, because this will reflect vastus-medialis obliques atrophy. The oblique head of the quadriceps vastus-medialis is often deficient and can best be observed in full extension.

Frequently associated with patellofemoral pain is tenderness about the inferior pole of the patella and along the patella tendon (Figure 5-5). This may be associated with the appearance of fragmentation of the inferior pole of the patella on the lateral x-ray that represents osteochondritis of the lower pole of the patella (Johansson-Larsen syndrome [39]). In the older patient who has fused his tibial apophysis, maximal stresses of running and jumping are exerted through the patella tendon to its insertion. Inflammation of the patella tendon, especially marked at the inferior pole of the patella tendon, is suggestive of "jumper's knee," or patella tendinitis [1].

Treatment of Patellofemoral Pain Syndrome
Once the diagnosis of patellofemoral pain syndrome has been established by history, physical examination, and appropriate x-ray studies, nonoperative treatment is started. The treatment protocol we use is based on the principles of Hughston, Allman, Collins, DeHaven, and others. It is divided into four phases:

1. Control of symptoms
2. Strengthening of quadriceps and hamstring muscles through isometric and isotonic progressive resistive exercises
3. A graduated running program
4. A maintenance program

Control of symptoms is obtained through rest and the avoidance of aggravating activities. Occasionally, the extremity must be immobilized in either a cylinder cast or knee immobilizer and crutches used. We also place the patient on aspirin, 10 gr, 4 times a day. There

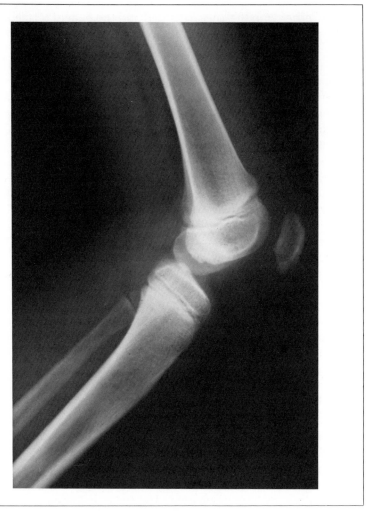

Figure 5-5. Fragmentation of the lower pole of the patella in a child with "jumper's knee."

is evidence to indicate that salicylates may inhibit cartilage degeneration [4].

As soon as the patient is able to tolerate them, the muscle strengthening exercises are begun. These are done once a day with 3 sets of 10 repetitions each. They may be performed with either a weighted exercise boot or an exercise machine. The quadriceps exercises are initially done isometrically doing straight leg lifts with the knee in full extension. It must be emphasized that extension is not to be performed actively against resistance through the range of motion because this will usually only aggravate the sypmtoms. In addition to the quadriceps isometric exercises, the patient does hamstring isotonic exercises through a range of motion. The appropriate ratio of quadricep to hamstring strengths is approximately 2 to 1.

Only when the symptoms are controlled does the patient begin a graduated running program. Generally, this occurs when the patient is able to do his quadriceps exercises with a 30-pound weight. The guidelines for exercises and running for a 175-pound male athlete are listed below. It should be noted that weight levels are modified according to the size of the patient.

Goal weights for quadriceps progressive resistive exercises:	Graduated running geared to quadriceps progressive resistive exercises:
30 pounds	Jogging
30–40 pounds	Half-speed running (straight ahead)
40–50 pounds	Three-quarter speed running
60 pounds	Full-speed running and cutting from side to side

A maintenance program is of utmost importance, and once the patient has achieved his desired weight and activity levels, he should continue exercising at therapeutic levels 2 to 3 times a week. Additionally, at this time, the patient may be fitted for shoe orthotics to correct pronation. A patella stabilizing brace, or cartilage brace, may help control subluxation. This brace consists of an elasticized cylinder with a hole cut out for the patella and medial and lateral stabilizing pads to help centralize the patella.

It is extremely important to encourage the patient during his course of nonoperative treatment. It has been our experience that greater than 80 percent of patients who follow this nonoperative program will be able to either resume unrestricted athletics with no disability during or after the activities, or resume restricted athletic activities without disability. We give nonoperative treatment a trial period of at least six months and only if it is then found to be ineffective do we recommend surgery.

The treatment for patella tendinitis must be preventive. Although it is difficult to stop an athlete who is only mildly affected from pursuing his sport, such restriction can usually prevent progression and aggravation of the problem. Antiinflammatory drugs such as aspirin, Butazolidin 100 mg 3 times a day after meals for 7 days, or Indocin 25 mg 3 times a day after meals may be helpful. Controversy exists concerning steroid injections about the patella tendon. Kennedy and Baxter–Willis [21] have shown that a tendon is significantly weakened for a period of 2 to 3 weeks following such an injection. It is no doubt best to avoid using steroid injections and it is absolutely contraindicated to inject directly into the tendon.

MENISCAL TEARS

Tears of the menisci have been reported in patients as early as the age of 5. They are more common in older adolescence. The typical history is that of locking, in which the knee has a mechanical block to flexion or extension [17]. The patient may have pain in the joint when an attempt is made to bring the knee to full flexion as in deep squatting. Physical examination may reveal a positive McMurray's circumduction test either medially or laterally, as well as tenderness along the joint line. If there is loss of range of motion, recurring symptoms, and a proven tear of the meniscus by arthrogram and/or arthroscopy, then menisectomy must be considered. The long-term effects of menisectomy in young children are not fully known. If there is associated ligamentous insufficiency, then menisectomy alone may produce increased joint laxity.

EPIPHYSEAL PLATE INJURIES

Although force applied to the lower extremity of a child is most often dissipated by fracture of the femur or tibia, occasionally, fractures occur through either the distal femoral or proximal tibial epiphyseal plates. These fractures account for 20 percent of all physeal injuries [39]. Epiphyseal plate injuries have been classified by Salter as Types I through V [36] (Figure 5-6). Type I occurs through the physis. Type II extends through the physis and out through the metaphysis. Type III transgresses the epiphysis and then extends along the physis. Type IV transgresses the epiphysis and the metaphysis. Type V represents a crushing injury. The distal femoral epiphysis contributes approximately 70 percent to the longitudinal growth of the femur and the proximal tibial epiphysis contributes approximately 60 percent to the total growth of the tibia. It is therefore extremely important to recognize fractures of these growth plates and treat them appropriately.

Physical examination may reveal tenderness about the growth plates, evidence of deformity, and excessive ligamentous laxity. In order to differentiate between ligament tears and epiphyseal fractures, it is frequently necessary to obtain stress x-rays. Once growth plate fractures are recognized, it is extremely important to follow appropriate treatment protocols. In general, Types I and II injuries have an excellent prognosis for prompt healing and no residual growth disturbances when managed by closed reduction and casting. Types III and IV injuries usually require open reduction and internal fixation and have a more guarded prognosis. Type V injuries are quite serious and may go unrecognized until late growth arrest occurs. The patient and the family must be informed that subsequent growth disturbances

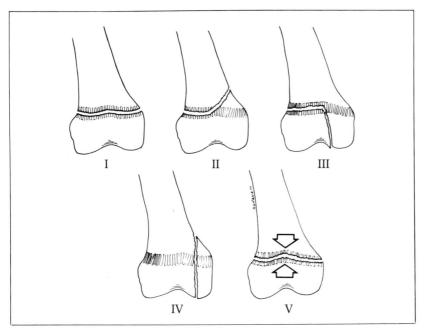

Figure 5-6. Salter classification of epiphyseal fractures.

can occur following such injuries. The patient should be followed for potential deformity formation until the end of growth.

LIGAMENTOUS INJURIES

As mentioned previously, although injury to ligaments of the knee in children less than 14 years old is unusual, such injuries do occur and one must maintain a high index of suspicion in order to diagnose them (see Figure 5-3). The anatomy of the knee is such that the origin and insertion of the collateral ligaments and joint capsule relative to the position of the femoral and tibial epiphyseal plates favor physeal disruption rather than damage to the ligaments, which are stronger than the growth plate. Following a standard history, physical examination, and roentgenograms, one may choose to aspirate the knee and inject local anesthetic in order to allow a more thorough examination. Occasionally, stress roentgenograms may be helpful. If there is any question, one should examine the knee under general anesthesia and obtain stress roentgenograms in the operating room. Additionally, arthroscopy of the knee may offer help in accurately defining the location and extent of intra-articular knee pathology [6].

Concomitant ligament injuries should be sought in patients found to have an avulsion of the tibial intercondylar eminence [5, 24, 25]. Avulsion of the tibial intercondylar eminence is usually associated with avulsion injury to the anterior cruciate ligament. A typical history is that of a 12-year-old child who falls off a bicycle and develops an acute painful hemarthrosis. Avulsion of the anterior cruciate ligament with the tibial spine must be considered the diagnosis until proven otherwise. If such an injury is diagnosed, treatment may be open or closed, depending on the degree of displacement of the tibial spine.

LEG INJURIES

Injuries to the leg in children and adolescents are either of the acute type due to a specific traumatic incident, or more insidious in nature secondary to overuse syndromes.

As has been pointed out previously, skiing is a sport in which acute fractures of the tibia are not all that uncommon in children. In Nilsson and Roass' review of soccer injuries in adolescents [29] there were only four fractures of the tibia and two depression fractures of the tibial condyle in 25,000 players who took part in 2,987 soccer matches. Although soccer is a relatively safe sport for adolescents, with a low injury rate, the biomechanics of kicking has been the subject of scientific analysis [11]. It should be realized that kicking involves the generation of large amounts of kinetic energy in lower extremities, and only part of this energy is transferred to the ball, the rest being dissipated by the leg in the follow-through. During the follow-through phase of kicking, the leg of the kicker becomes vulnerable to injury by other players, while the moving leg itself becomes a dangerous missile that can inflict severe injury. Although the actual incidence of tibial fracture and knee injuries due to kicking is low, we must consider injury prevention in the sport. Indeed, when one thinks of the biomechanics of kicking and looks at the adult size, number 5 soccer ball that has become considerably heavier as it is played on a wet surface, there seems little doubt that it would be prudent to insist on the use of the smaller number 3 or 4 balls by the smaller children. This would no doubt lower the stresses imparted to the growing structures of the lower extremities.

OVERUSE SYNDROMES

The young athlete is particularly prone to overuse syndromes. Two of the most common are stress fractures and shin splints. Orada and Saarela [32] studied the nature of exertion injuries that occurred in young athletes who had started extensive sports training at an early age. With puberty, growth disorders, sudden growth spurts, changes in body structure, and motor coordination cause problems to both the athletes and the coaches. The ideal patterns of loading and optimum stresses to which the growing child should be subjected are not yet clearly defined, and it is still difficult to prescribe the exact amount, intensity, and frequency of different training sessions for young athletes in particular sports.

Of the exertion injuries observed by Orada and Saarela, one-third were orthopedic pain syndromes typical for the growing age, while two-thirds were typical of exertion injuries seen in older athletes. Of those problems classified as actual sports injuries, muscle compartment ischemic pain in the legs, stress fractures, and insertion tendonopathies such as achilles tendinitis were the most difficult to treat and took the longest time to heal. Acute injuries of the leg included muscle rupture in the leg, heel bruise, and ligament injuries of the ankle. Orthopedic problems of the young athletes that occurred were calcaneal apophysitis, Osgood–Schlatter's disease, Achilles tendon peribursitis, muscle pain in the calf, stress fracture of the fibula, and patella tendinitis. It must be emphasized that in young children and adolescent athletes, prevention of exertion injuries is especially important and great care must be taken in paying enough attention to symptoms, when educating coaches and trainers, and to acquiring a knowledge and understanding of young people's exertion injuries. As would be expected, the risk of injury is smallest in supervised and guided sports activities [19].

STRESS FRACTURES

A stress fracture is a break in a bone, either partial or complete, secondary to submaximal cyclic loading. It may, therefore, be thought of as a process rather then as a single traumatic event. During repetitive loading of the respective bone, the body's rate of healing eventually is overwhelmed and the bone fractures. The classic history is that of gradual onset of pain in the area of the fracture at the end of the activity session. The pain is usually relieved by rest but when the activity is resumed it is noticed that the pain evolves into an ache and occurs nearer to the onset of the exercise. Eventually, the pain begins as soon as the exercise starts and rest does not relieve the pain. In fact, the pain may awaken the athlete at night. This cycle of events may take anywhere from a few days to several months.

Physical examination usually reveals an area of tenderness over the lesion, with slight periosteal reaction and sclerosis at the area of the fracture. Walter and Wolff have found the proximal tibial metaphysis to be the most common site of stress fractures in young athletes [42]. Devas differentiated between adult and juvenile forms of stress fractures [8]. The juvenile form occurs in cancellous bone with compression stress applied to the trabecular bone. Apparently, microfracture of the trabeculae is followed by an osteoblastic reparative process and one sees internal callus formation without the presence of a lucent line on the x-ray (Figure 5-7). The adult variety, on the other hand, occurs more commonly in cortical bone areas and may represent a

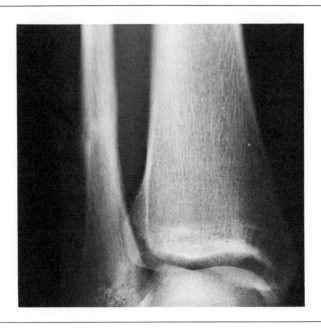

Figure 5-7. Stress fracture of the distal fibula in a young runner.

failure in tension in which a lucent line appears prior to evidence of osteoblastic repair. In addition to the proximal tibia, stress fractures do occur in other bones in young athletes. They have been reported in the fibula, in patients as young as 2 years of age. It is important to emphasize that a high index of suspicion is frequently necessary to make the appropriate diagnosis when faced with a patient complaining of rather vague symptoms. All too frequently the combination of a rather vague history with negative x-rays in an emotional teenager results in attributing the problem to a psychogenic origin.

SHIN SPLINTS

This is a condition frequently associated with running or jogging. Although the usual onset is insidious, it may develop into severe discomfort that may interfere with performance. Typically, tenderness is felt along the inside (posteriomedial) border of the tibia. This site corresponds to the tibialis posterior muscle origin. Although the mechanism of injury is unknown, it may represent repeated small tears at the site of the origin of the posterior tibial muscle from the tibia and the interosseous membrane between the tibia and the fibula. X-ray examination usually is normal. Sometimes, involvement of the anterior tibial muscle at the anterior border of the tibia and onto its anterolateral face is also called "shin splints," although this may actually represent a compartmental compression syndrome.

Considerations in differential diagnosis would be stress fracture of the tibia, compartmental ischemic compression syndrome, and muscle tear. Tenderness in the stress fracture is generally more localized and there may be positive roentgenographic findings. Compartmental compression syndromes occur frequently in the anterior compartment of the leg where the tibialis anterior muscle is surrounded by non-yielding fascia. Compartmental compression syndrome symptoms generally occur during exercise or following exercise and are often associated with tingling, numbness, and loss of motor strength. It is now possible to perform percutaneous pressure measurements of the intracompartmental pressure that helps confirm the diagnosis of compression syndrome. Treatment for the compression syndrome generally requires fasciotomy. Muscle tears, such as in the medial head of the gastrocnemius, often have an acute history in which the patient feels a specific sudden onset of pain. There may be associated hemorrhage and a defect in the muscle.

The treatment of shin splints involves resting the part and the use of local ice. Adhesive tape strapping of the foot to relieve stress on the posterior tibial muscle may give marked improvement. It is frequently necessary to run on a softer surface and to change running shoes to a type which has a more shock-absorbing sole. Resumption of activity must be carefully supervised to avoid recurrence. The physical examination must pay particular attention to foot alignment and, if necessary, foot orthotics may have to be prescribed to prevent excessive pronation and subsequent stress on the posterior tibial muscle. Emphasis must be placed on accurate diagnosis so that one may treat a specific condition rather than one subsumed under the general term "shin splints."

ANKLE AND FOOT INJURIES

Children can sustain ligamentous sprains to the ankle as do adults. However, one must be alert to the possibility of epiphyseal fractures and growth plate injuries in both the tibia and fibula. Although x-ray examinations may be interpreted as normal, tenderness and soft tissue swelling about the distal fibula epiphysis must be considered a Salter–Harris Type I injury and treated with appropriate immobilization in a short leg cast. Permanent damage and deformity to the ankle joint can occur if growth in the distal fibula ceases because of injury. In the differential diagnosis, osteochondral fractures in the ankle, especially the talus, must be considered when there is pain and swelling that persist in an otherwise stable ankle that has been recently injured.

The child is also prone to apophyseal avulsion injuries, particularly at the base of the fifth metatarsal, where the peroneus brevis tendon inserts. Avulsion of the base of the fifth metatarsal may occur with forced, unexpected inversion in an everted foot. The prognosis is good and the injury responds well either to protected weight-bearing and a gentle compressive wrap, or to a short cast. This avulsion must be differentiated from a fracture through the proximal diaphysis of the fifth metatarsal that may go on to nonunion requiring bone grafting, despite adequate treatment in a cast.

Irritation of the calcaneal apophysis in the area of insertion of the Achilles tendon may occur. Pain and tenderness about the posterior calcaneaus associated with a dense apophysis on x-ray is known as Sever's disease or calcaneal apophysitis. It should be noted, however, that increased density of the calcaneal apophysitis is frequently a finding in asymptomatic children. When one is faced with heelcord and calcaneal apophyseal pain syndrome, the child must be evaluated for heelcord tightness. It may be necessary that appropriate stretching activities of the gastrocnemius and soleus muscle complex be instituted. Additional treatment measures include the use of aspirin and intermittent icing. Occasionally, a short cast is necessary to immobilize the extremity for about two weeks until the symptoms subside. Immobilization must be followed by stretching and muscle strengthening exercises, so that symmetrical strength and full range of motion are regained prior to resumption of activity.

REFERENCES

1. Blazina, M. E., et al.   Jumper's knee. *Orthop. Clin. North Am.* 4:665, 1973.
2. Bergfeld, J.   First-, second-, and third-degree sprains. *Am. J. Sports Med.* 7:207, 1979.
3. Cahill, B. R.   Stress fractures of the proximal tibial epiphysis: A case report. *Am. J. Sports Med.* 5:180, 1977.
4. Chrisman, D. D., and Snook, G. A.   The role of patelloplasty and patellectomy in the arthritic knee. *Clin. Orthop.* 101:40, 1974.
5. Clanton, T., et al.   Knee ligament injuries in children. *J. Bone Joint Surg. [Am.].* 61A:1195, 1979.
6. DeHaven, K. E.   Diagnosis of acute knee injuries with hemarthrosis. *Am. J. Sports Med.* 8:8, 1980.
7. DeHaven, K. E., Dolan, W., and Mayer, P.   Chondromalacia patella and the painful knee. *Am. Fam. Physician* 21:117, 1980.
8. Devas, M.   *Stress Fractures.* London: Churchill Livingstone, 1975.
9. Eilert, R. E.   Sports injuries in children. *Surg. Rounds* 1:54, 1978.
10. Eriksson, E.   Reconstruction of the anterior cruciate ligament. *Orthop. Clin. North Am.* 7:167, 1976.
11. Gainor, B. J., et al.   The kick biomechanics and collison injury. *Am. J. Sports Med.* 6:185, 1978.
12. Galway, R. D.   Pivot shift syndrome. *J. Bone Joint Surg. [Br].* 54:558, 1972.
13. Galway, R. D., Beaupre, A., and MacIntosh, D. L.   Pivot shift, a clinical sign of symptomatic anterior cruciate insufficiency. *J. Bone Joint Surg. [Br.]* 54:763, 1972.

14. Garrick, J. G., and Requa, R. H.   Injury patterns in children and adolescent skiers. *Am. J. Sports Med.* 7:245, 1979.
15. Godshall, R. W.   Junior league football: risks versus benefits. *Am. J. Sports Med.* 3:139, 1975.
16. Green, W. T., and Banks, H. E.   Osteochondritis dissecans in children. *J. Bone Joint Surg. [Am.]* 35:26, 1953.
17. Grossman, R., and Nicholas, J.   Common disorders of the knee. *Orthop. Clin. North Am.* 8:619, 1977.
18. James, S.   Chondromalacia of the Patella in the Adolescent. In J. C. Kennedy (Ed.), *The Injured Adolescent Knee.* Baltimore: Williams & Wilkins, 1979.
19. James, S. L., Bates, B., and Osternig, L. R.   Injuries to runners. *Am. J. Sports Med.* 6:40, 1978.
20. Kennedy, J. C. (Ed.).   *The Injured Adolescent Knee.* Baltimore: Williams & Wilkins, 1979.
21. Kennedy, J. C., and Baxter-Willis, R.   The effects of local steriod injections on tendons: A biomechanical and microscopic correlative study. *Am. J. Sports Med.* 4:11, 1976.
22. Marshall, J. L., and Rubin, R.   Knee ligament injuries—diagnostic and therapeutic approach. *Orthop. Clin. North Am.* 8:641, 1977.
23. Mayer, R. J., and Micheli, L. J.   Avulsion of the femoral attachment of the posterior cruciate ligament in an 11-year-old boy. *J. Bone Joint Surg. [Am.]* 61:431, 1979.
24. Meyers, M. H., and McKeever, F. M.   Fractures of the intercondylar eminence of the tibia. *J. Bone Joint Surg. [Am.]* 41:209, 1959.
25. Meyers, M. H., and McKeever, F. M.   Fractures of the intercondylar eminence of the tibia. *J. Bone Joint Surg. [Am.]* 52:1677, 1970.
26. Micheli, L. J.   Sports Injuries in Children and Adolescents. In R. H. Strauss (Ed.), *Sports Medicine and Physiology.* Philadelphia: Saunders, 1979. P. 289.
27. Mital, M. A., and Mitza, R. A.   Osgood Schlatter's disease: the painful puzzler. *Physicians Sports Med.* 5:60, 1977.
28. Neiss Report, National Electronic Injury Surveillance System. U.S. Consumer Product Safety Commission, May 1976–May 1977. Washington, D.C.: U.S. Government Printing Office, 1978.
29. Nilsson, S., and Roass, A.   Soccer injuries in adolescents. *Am. J. Sports Med.* 6:358, 1978.
30. O'Donoghue, D. H.   End result of knee ligament surgery. *J. Bone Joint Surg. [Am.]* 37:1, 1955.
31. O'Donoghue, D. H.   *The Treatment of Injuries in Athletes.* Philadelphia: Saunders, 1976.
32. Orava, S., and Saarela, J.   Exertion injuries to young athletes. *Am. J. Sports Med.* 6:68, 1978.
33. Quigley, T. B.   Common Muscular Skeletal Problems. In R. H. Strauss (Ed.), *Sports Medicine and Physiology.* Philadelphia: Saunders, 1979.
34. Roberts, J.   Osteochondritis Dissecans. In J. C. Kennedy (Ed.), *The Injured Adolescent Knee.* Baltimore: Williams & Wilkins, 1979.
35. Roser, L. A., and Clawson, D. K.   Football injuries in the very young athletes. *Clin. Orthop.* 69:212, 1970.
36. Salter, R. B., and Harris, W. R.   Injuries involving the epiphyseal plate. *J. Bone Joint Surg. [Am.]* 45:587, 1963.
37. Saunders, W., Wilkins, K., and Neidre, A.   Acute insufficiency of the posterior cruciate ligament in children. *J. Bone Joint Surg. [Am.]* 62:129, 1980.

38. Sharrard, W.   *Pediatric Orthopaedics and Fractures.* Oxford, Engl.: Blackwell, 1971. P. 400.
39. Tachdjian, M. O.   *Pediatric Orthopaedics.* Philadelphia: Saunders, 1972. Pp. 1706-1719.
40. Tapper, E. M.   Ski injuries from 1939 to 1976: the Sun Valley experience. *Am. J. Sports Med.* 6:114, 1978.
41. Torg, J. S., Conrad, W., and Kalen, V.   Clinical diagnosis of anterior cruciate ligament instability in the athlete. *Am. J. Sports Med.* 4:84, 1976.
42. Walter, M., and Wolf, M.   Stress fractures in young athletes. *Am. J. Sports Med.* 5:165, 1977.

6. Spinal Injuries in Children's Sports

Douglas W. Jackson

Injuries to the spine and adjacent soft tissue in the child athlete are usually associated with short periods of disability. Spinal damage with permanent sequelae is infrequent, but the possibility does exist for quite serious injury. Fractures or dislocations of the boney column, with or without associated neurological damage, represent the most severe end of the spectrum of spinal injuries that can occur in the childhood athlete. The child's spine has the good healing and restorative capabilities of youth, but in the remaining growth potential lies the possibility of accentuating certain deformities. Thus, spinal injuries in the child deserve special attention and may require special experience in treating them.

PREVENTING SPINAL INJURIES

At the present time there is no good protective equipment for the young athlete that will prevent spinal trauma. Effective protection for the head is provided for by different forms of protective helmets, but nothing to date has been developed to protect the cervical, thoracic, or lumbar spine from potential injuries. The helmet may protect the head in certain sports, technique and chance protect the spine.

Spinal injuries in children can be reduced primarily by minimizing the exposure to high-risk situations. Sports and activities that increase the speed that the child is able to attain, that place the child at heights where he or she can fall, or place him or her in jeopardy of being struck by an automobile are of particularly high risk, e.g., hang-gliding, bicycling, roller-skating or skateboarding in traffic, or inappropriate use of motorcycles. Spinal injuries can be minimized by adhering to the rules governing the activity and the teaching of proper form and technique. It is of particular importance in sports such as gymnastics, diving, equestrian events, and other potentially high-risk sports that the youngster be directed in an orderly and step-wise fashion to the development of skill levels adequate to the more difficult and dangerous maneuvers. Coaching, supervision of practice periods, safe facilities, and proper use and maintenance of equipment are also important elements in the reduction of spinal injuries in children. However, even with careful attention to detail, spinal injuries will occur and certain sports will have a higher incidence of potentially devastating spinal injuries.

ACUTE SPINAL INJURIES

The treatment of acute spinal trauma emergencies will not be covered in detail within this chapter. However, the physician should be able to recognize and triage the severe spinal injuries that occur unexpectedly. This is best done by giving forethought to the possibility of such an injury and becoming familiar with various types of immobilization and transportation techniques, the locations of treatment facilities, and specialists and specialized care. Severe injuries may occur in remote locations (e.g., when rock-climbing or mountaineering) or close to medical facilities. Such sports as motorcycling, hang-gliding, diving, football, roller-skating, skateboarding, surfing, skiing, bicycling, and gymnastics provide settings that can be quite different. The initial evaluation and triage may call upon the resources of those persons immediately available for care.

There are certain principles in caring for spinal injuries occurring in the athlete that each physician should be familiar with. They include:

1. Be calm, the initial injury has occurred.
2. Prevent any extension of the spinal injury and prevent a secondary injury by proper protection, immobilization, and transportation.
3. Triage the youngster to an appropriate medical facility safely.
4. When possible communicate the initial findings and care rendered with the physician assuming responsibility. The definitive diagnosis, treatment, and rehabilitation should be rendered by appropriate specialists and medical centers.

In addition to recognizing spinal trauma in the conscious child, the unconscious young athlete deserves the following special considerations: *a.* A youngster rendered unconscious as the result of a direct blow should be treated as a cervical injury until proven otherwise. *b.* In the unconscious patient, the protective headgear need not be removed. It is not urgent to remove the headgear unless in some way it is interfering with adequate ventilation of the patient. *c.* If removal is necessary take great care in removing the fitted headgear with strap fixation under the chin from the athlete who is unconscious. Subjecting the cervical spine to additional movement may cause an associated injury. Where possible, the unconscious athlete, and the athlete with a cervical spine injury, should be transported in their helmet, or other equipment, by the safest means. This does not apply when trauma has not been the cause of the unconsciousness.

Evaluating the stability of an acute spinal injury can best be done in an emergency room or clinic where roentgenograms are available. Adequate roentgenographic evaluation can be difficult to obtain because of the immobility of the child with a spinal injury. In those cases in which spinal films of the injured area are inadequate one must highly suspect a significant injury. It is after the boney structure of the spine has been demonstrated to be intact and aligned appropriately that different methods may be used for determining ligamentous stability. Confirmation of spinal stability may require further testing if it is felt to be necessary.

DIAGNOSES

The diagnostic tests used for children and teenagers in the evaluation of spinal injuries, or pain-producing lesions of the spine, are similar to those studies used for the adult. In addition to a careful history and physical examination, studies usually include routine roentgenograms. Special roentgenographic views to accentuate certain areas of the spine, conventional tomography, computerized axial tomography, bone scans, venograms, myelograms, electromyograms and cineradiography may be used selectively in certain cases. Supplemental diagnostic tests are seldom necessary, as most processes associated with spinal pain and injuries are self-limiting, benign processes that represent a straightforward diagnosis.

Unexplained spinal pain that persists in the youngster needs to be explained and pursued in great detail. It may possibly be a manifestation of a more subtle injury, but occasionally neoplasms may present in association with athletic injuries. Although they are rare, tumors involving the boney, neural, or adjacent soft tissue in the spine should not be overlooked. Those that develop slowly may be quite difficult to diagnose, particularly when the young athlete attributes the onset of pain to an athletic activity or participation. In the young and developing child, thinking of the spinal column as a unit is helpful in the evaluation of injury. Restricted motion secondary to tight paraspinous soft-tissue structures, or certain boney abnormalities resulting in restricted motion of segments of the spine, need special assessment.

The majority of childhood spinal injuries that result in chronic pain are confined to the thoracic and lumbar spine and are often the result of repetitive, noncatastrophic injuries. These include sprains and strains, subtle fractures, stress fractures, growth plate injuries, disc injuries, and developmental structural changes. These chronic situations often follow injuries in which adequate time for healing has not been allowed, contributing to the chronicity of the problem. The potential for healing is delayed by continued participation in aggravating activities. The subsequent alterations of the healing process may be associated with pain and secondary chronic changes.

Early rehabilitation is possible and desirable even following quite severe spinal injury. The young athlete, following spinal injuries resulting in associated instability such as a fracture/subluxation of the cervical spine, responds nicely to rigid fixation and early ambulation. The halo-jacket fixation is quite an effective means of immobilizing the head and cervical spine. It can be coupled either with surgery or nonsurgical treatment of cervical injuries. Special bracing can also be used following the thoracic and lumbar spine injury in most cases to allow for early ambulation of the young athlete.

Normal range of motion and excursion of the entire spine will prevent some injuries and relieve some of the discomfort the youngster may experience when participating in repetitive activities that require the extremes of spinal motion. Stretching should be part of the youngster's warmup and training, particularly in sports requiring repetitive use of the spine. Such obvious sports are gymnastics and weightlifting, but even running involves repetitive motion of the lumbar spine. There are few sports that children participate in seriously in which the child would not be benefited by doing spinal stretching exercises.

THORACIC SPINE

The thoracic spine differs from the cervical and lumbar spine in that the presence of a rib cage results in a more restricted range of motion for the thoracic spine and seems to protect it, leaving the cervical and lumbar spine more susceptible to the more catastrophic injuries.

Compression fractures of the vertebral bodies and end-plate fractures in the thoracic spine in young athletes should be suspected. These compression fractures may be easily recognizable if the vertebral bodies' usual roentgenographic shape is altered, but they may also be associated with minimal boney compression. A boney injury with only a disruption of the vertebral end-plate, or minimal compression, may be overlooked on routine roentgenograms. Those youngsters that have thoracic pain of a greater or more persistent nature should be suspected of having a boney component to their injury, particularly if associated with thoracic paraspinous muscle spasm and guarding. Some boney injuries may be demonstrated only by sequential roentgenograms, or by obtaining a positive technetium pyrophosphate bone scan. Increased vertebral activity on the bone scan becomes detectable within 3 to 5 days of a boney injury to the spine in the young athlete. The scan may demonstrate increased osteoblastic activity in relationship to a spinal trauma. This allows the physician, in certain cases, to prescribe a longer period of immobilization and rest to allow for adequate healing.

During active growth spurts spinal deformities may require restrictive bracing. This bracing may place restrictions on certain sports activities. However, fitness and maintenance of flexibility remain an important part of the treatment. Those youngsters with compensated curves and who maintain spinal flexibility are not significantly handicapped in athletic participation. Complete thoracic range of motion and the stretching out of tight paraspinous soft-tissue structures have been important in those athletes involved in sports requiring repetitive, strenuous use of the entire spine. An example of this is gymnastics where time is spent increasing and maintaining range of motion in the thoracic spine as well as throughout the entire spine.

Scheuermann's Disease

Scheuermann's disease, or juvenile kyphosis, is less frequently seen in the young athletic population although it has been felt by some that repetitive trauma is a possible etiology [1, 7, 8, 9]. The anterior vertebral wedging of three or more vertebral bodies is necessary to make this diagnosis. The round-back deformity that may develop is often not associated with pain. The child is usually initially brought for evaluation because of concern over the child's posture. The primary-care physician should refer the youngsters that are more involved, as well as those showing signs of progression and significant roentgenographic changes.

Scoliosis

Scoliosis is another entity involving the thoracic spine that may alter the posture of the developing child. It is often detected by associated changes manifested in the rib cage and unusual curvature in the thoracic spine. Scoliosis is not a contraindication to participation in sports by the young athlete (Figure 6-1). Many top-level national and international athletes have competed successfully with scoliosis. Ideally, if scoliosis is picked up at a young age and referred for appropriate evaluation and treatment, very few of the young athletes will be severely restricted by this condition. Scoliosis is not the result of spinal trauma as best understood at this point. The occurrence of scoliosis is more frequent in young women. In general, it does not preclude the youngster from athletic enjoyment and participation.

Traumatic Anterior Disc Herniation

Traumatic anterior disc herniation through the ring apophysis as the result of trauma should not be confused with Scheuermann's disease (Figure 6-2A, B, C). This traumatic injury is not associated with vertebral wedging in terms of the anterior height of the vertebral body. There is no undulation of the vertebral end-plate and the condition does not progress to give a round-back deformity. Although this entity can be associated with pain and can restrict athletic participation for a period of time, it is usually self-limiting. The disc space narrowing usually involves the lower thoracic and upper lumbar area and is most often seen at the thoracolumbar junction. Bracing may be indicated. Protection of the area from repetitive trauma may even be associated with some restoration of the disc space. Participation in athletics usually remains possible. Only the more severe cases during the painful phase may need some restriction.

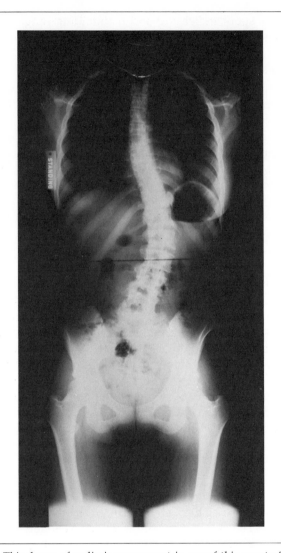

Figure 6-1. This degree of scoliosis was present in one of this country's top-level female gymnasts. She maintained good flexibility in spite of these structural changes.

Figure 6-2. (A)Anterior disc herniation at the T$_{12}$–L$_1$ disc space with secondary changes on apophyseal development of the first lumbar vertebra. Note significant disc space narrowing in this 15-year-old wrestler. Also, less apparent on the lateral view is the presence of bilateral L$_5$ pars interarticularis defects. (B) Note distinct changes at two vertebral levels in this young gymnast. (C) Diagrammatic representation of Schmorl's description of this traumatic protrusion of the nucleus pulposus in the young athlete.

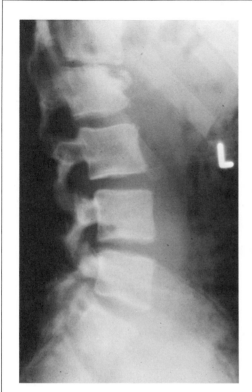

A

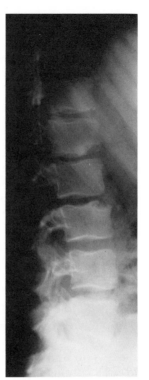

B

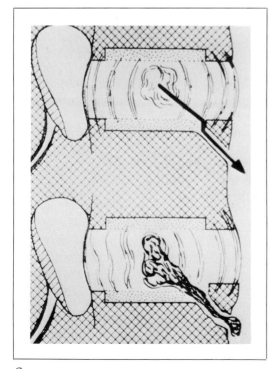

C

LUMBAR SPINE

Because of the increasing number of young people participating in highly competitive, year-round, structured athletics, more athletes are presenting with complaints of chronic low back pain [2]. The physician confronted with a preteen or adolescent athlete with a low back pain or injury has to establish a diagnosis, start an appropriate treatment, and indicate to the youngster when he or she will be able to resume participation in competitive sports.

The significance of lumbar pain varies in the young athlete. The more common entities resulting in chronic pain that interferes with athletic performance include:

1. Soft tissue injuries, not allowed time for healing, including sprains and strains
2. Stress reactions of the posterior elements—the pars interarticularis
3. Spondylolisthesis
4. End-plate fracures of the vertebral bodies
5. Symptomatic lumbar disc injuries

There is no convincing evidence that any type of treatment for the child with chronic low back pain is superior to nature's own course, if rest and prevention of re-injury are allowed over a period of time. This does not apply, of course, to back pain resulting from neoplasm or structural instability such as spondylolisthesis.

SOFT TISSUE INJURY

Soft tissue injuries involving musculotendonous units, ligaments, and periarticular structures are usually not isolated, but occur in combination. A specific diagnosis in the child is usually not necessary. These injuries respond rapidly to rest (absolute or partial) and prevention of extension of the injury. Recovery from the majority of soft tissue injuries usually takes 1 to 3 weeks, after which pain-free participation may be resumed. It is important to maintain conditioning and flexibility within this disability period without aggravating the pain. Antilordotic positioning and exercises are usually indicated and hyperextension of the spine should be avoided. This may vary depending on the mechanism of injury.

Bracing young athletes for soft tissue injuries is usually not necessary and can be negatively associated with disuse muscle atrophy. If bracing is felt to be necessary to slow the patient down, an antilordotic brace may be most beneficial (Figure 6-3). The brace can be removed for therapy, stretching and exercise. Therapy progresses according to pain. No treatment has yet been documented that hastens the healing process in the lumbar spine in soft tissue injuries faster than rest and avoiding aggravation and re-injury.

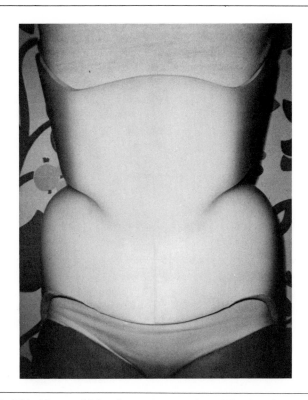

Figure 6-3. This 11-year-old female gymnast was immobilized with the lower portion of the Boston Brace. The antilordotic posture and its help as a reminder to restrict activity have been useful in certain low back problems in young athletes.

STRESS REACTIONS

The typical presentation of a developing stress reaction in the posterior elements of the lumbar spine is with a youngster with an aching low back pain (usually unilateral), which is exaggerated by motion, particularly twisting and hyperextension [3, 4, 12]. Almost all such children have less pain in the reclining or supine position. Neurologic deficits and nerve root tension signs are uniformly absent in this entity. The pain is demonstrated and reproduced by the standing one-legged hyperextension maneuver. This test is not pathognomic, but does indicate posterior element irritation.

The history is usually one of vigorous participation in a sport requiring repetitive use of the low back and is often associated with jarring activities from such sports as gymnastics, football, wrestling, weight lifting, karate, pole-vaulting, and hurdling. Roentgenograms of the lumbar spine are often initially negative. Early confirmation of a boney reaction can be made with a positive technetium pyrophos-

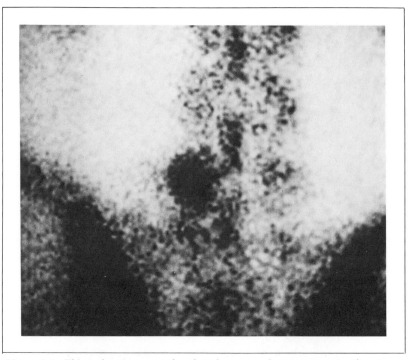

Figure 6-4. This technetium pyrophosphate bone scan demonstrates significant unilateral uptake in the posterior element of L_5 in this young pitcher. High resolution columnation on oblique views is often necessary to confirm the location of the increased uptake of the radioactive isotope.

phate bone scan (Figure 6-4). The bone scan has been shown to be a highly useful diagnostic and management tool in establishing or ruling out this entity. Recognition and early treatment of this boney injury may prevent the development of the pars interarticularis defect and may hasten the patient's return to his or her previous endeavors. The return to a normal condition on the bone scan tends to correlate closely with the abatement of the young athlete's symptoms.

PARS INTERARTICULARIS DEFECTS

The stress defects developing in a competitive athlete seem to differ from the pars interarticularis defects that appear in early childhood. The pars interarticularis defects that develop between the ages of 5 and 8 tend to arise out of a more significant hereditary predisposition, have associated dysplasia of adjacent posterior elements (e.g., spina bifida occulta), and tend to develop without pain or any symptomatic findings.

The athlete developing pars interarticularis defects usually does so without a high propensity to vertebral slippage (Figure 6-5). Very few

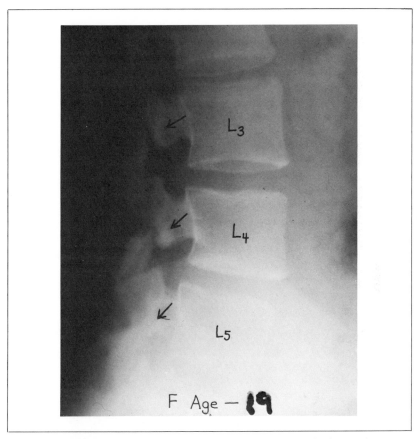

Figure 6-5. This young equestrian had intermittent, recurring back pain during her adolescent years. Multiple level pars interarticularis defects are often associated with segmental instability. This altered motion can often be demonstrated with flexion and extension views of cineradiography.

of these athletic youngsters go on to more than Grade I spondylo-listhesis if slippage does occur. The main objectives in treatment are the early recognition of this problem and the restriction of the activity associated with the back pain. Prevention of the development of a positive roentgenographic finding in the pars interarticularis defect is desirable, but is not always necessary to achieve relief of pain (Figure 6-6).

The time it takes to return to pain-free activity once the youngster develops a positive bone scan may vary anywhere from 6 weeks to 2 years, and is related, of course, to allowing adequate time for healing and rehabilitation. Treatment may be hastened by the use of some type of molded antilordotic brace to restrict lumbar motion, in particular hyperextension of the lumbar spine.

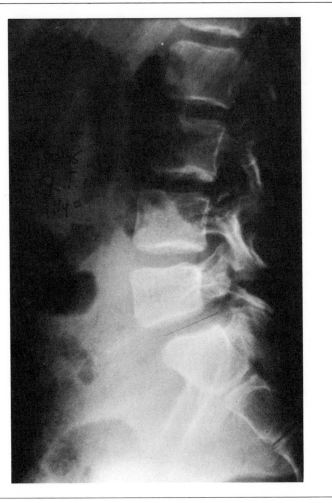

Figure 6-6. Asymptomatic Grade I spondylolisthesis in a top-level 11-year-old female gymnast. Incidental finding at the time of a low back survey in young female gymnasts.

SPONDYLOLISTHESIS

Spondylolisthesis is derived from the Greek *spondylo* meaning "spine" and *olisthesis* meaning "to slip or slide down a slippery path" [10, 11]. In the athlete we are basically talking about low grades of vertebral slippage of 50 percent or less. The majority of athletes who have spondylolisthesis have Grade I slippage and a minimal segmental instability. Youngsters with pars defects, without vertebral slippage, and those with vertebral slippage of less than 50 percent, are usually able to participate in all sports pain-free, or with only minimal intermittent restrictions.

The incidence of high-degree vertebral slippage is at least twice as high in girls as boys, yet the actual incidence of pars interarticularis defects has traditionally been higher in boys. However, this is changing in the athletic female population where there is now seen an increasing incidence of such defects in those young girls participating in strenuous sports demanding use of the lumbar spine. The youngster who goes on to high-degree slippage tends to be the nonathletic female.

The typical youngster with a high degree of slip will show the typical spondylolisthesis build with a short torso, heart-shaped flat buttocks, a rib cage that appears low, iliac crests that appear high, and a vertical

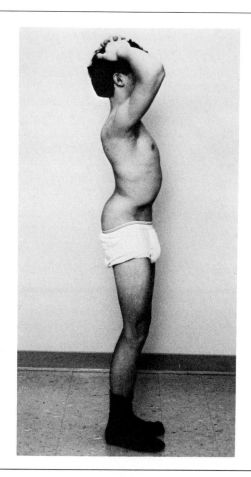

Figure 6-7. A vertical sacrum, shortened torso, and tight hamstrings are apparent in this young male with a high degree of spondylolisthesis. He has bilateral pars interarticularis defects at the L_5 vertebra. (Patient of Dr. Leon Wiltse.)

sacrum (Figure 6-7). The gait is altered by the tight hamstrings and, because of the vertical sacrum, the hips do not fully extend. A sciatic scoliosis may be present in high-degree vertebral slippage. The age of greatest vertebral slippage is between 9 and 14. Once the youngster is skeletally mature, further slippage is minimal.

The treatment of high-degree vertebral slippage presents a distinct isolated problem and the segments may be fused in situ, or reduced with instrumentation and then fused. For those patients with spondylolisthesis and chronic, recurrent low back pain, a lumbar fusion at the level of the segments' instability may be beneficial. Fusion can be done, and has been done, successfully in returning young athletes to pain-free competition. Several things need to be contemplated in determining if the young athlete should have surgery. One needs to demonstrate that the roentgenographic defect and vertebral slippage are the source of pain. The athlete should be having enough trouble independent of the sport to merit the risk of such major surgery. Often the young athlete who has a spinal fusion and has invested the time in the one-year layoff usually associated with the fusion and post-operative course elects not to return to his or her previous sport.

Most athletes with spondylolisthesis with low degrees of slippage are performing and many are unaware of their condition. Successful participation in vigorous athletics with greater than 50 percent vertebral slippage is difficult because of the secondary structural changes such as sacral tilt and hamstring tightness. The youngster who elects to compete in vigorous sports and has a high degree of vertebral slippage seen in long-term followup tends to have significantly more trouble. However, the youngster with high-degree slippage may have had difficulty even if he or she had not participated in sports.

END-PLATE FRACTURES

End-plate fractures of vertebral bodies do occur (as described by Schmorl [8]) in the lumbar spine with a low incidence in young athletes. They are most frequently found at the T_{12} to L_1 levels. These fractures should not be confused with Scheuermann's disease. They are the traumatic occurrence of a herniation of the disc through the anterior portion of the vertebral body and growth plate and occur in a fairly localized area. They may be associated with transient pain and chronic changes related to the disc space. End-plate fractures are best understood as a process that usually involves less than three vertebrae. There usually is no significant anterior vertebral wedging or appreciable kyphosis on clinical examination. Once again, sufficient rest to allow healing to occur, or, on rare occasions, supplemental bracing, is usually satisfactory treatment.

LUMBAR DISC INJURIES

The most frequently diagnosed disc herniation in the young athlete is that associated with posterior lateral herniation affecting the adjacent neural elements and giving nerve root tension signs with the dermatomal distribution of pain into the lower extremity (referred to as "sciatica") [5, 6] (Figure 6-8).

The young athlete with a symptomatic lumbar disc requires surgery in only a small percentage of cases. Usually less than 20 percent of the teenagers presenting with acute sciatica go on to significant diagnostic evaluation and a consideration of surgery. The majority respond quite rapidly to bed rest; their symptoms come on rapidly and resolve rapidly. It should be noted that young athletes may return quite successfully to competition with or without disc surgery. However, once the young athlete has experienced prolonged irritation of the neural elements, he or she may never return to a previous performance level, and tolerance for an activity may be decreased. The young athlete often has to select another sport, or a less demanding position in the same sport. Chronic changes may persist even after

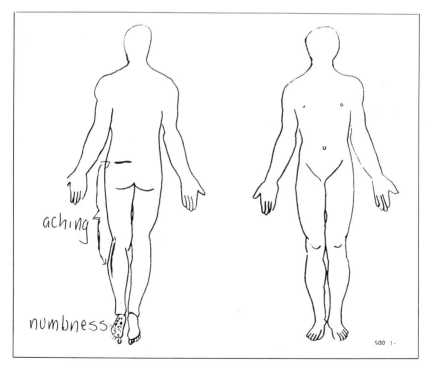

Figure 6-8. Asking the young athlete to draw where his or her pain is and to characterize it is a helpful technique in evaluating radiating pain.

successful lumbar surgical decompression of the extruded disc material. Intervertebral disc injuries in the young athlete may represent a one-level problem, or be the early presentation of a more chronic generalized lumbar disc problem.

NONSPECIFIC LOW BACK PAIN

A certain number of young athletes present with chronic low back pain associated with vigorous athletic participation. Physical examination, roentgenograms, a bone scan, and nerve root tension signs may all be interpreted as normal. These athletes may not be able to return to pain-free competition, even following the most sophisticated tests and consultations. The young people are relatively pain-free when not participating, but have pain with the vigorous demands of a given sport. Often after 6 months to 1 year of rest they can resume their sport without ever having had a specific diagnosis being confirmed. At times, selective bracing, coupled with stretching and strengthening exercises for the entire spine and limitation of their activities, will allow them to return sooner. Proper form and use of the low back in sports need to be evaluated by expert coaches and incorporated into the child's training routine. A careful assessment of flexibility and muscle balance may suggest certain strengthening exercises and a specific stretching and flexibility program.

Some youngsters may have a genetic propensity for the sero-negative spondyloarthropathies. Serologic studies like the HLA-B27 and others in the future may give us more insight. At the present time lumbar and "sacroilitic" discomfort as the result of an underlying spondyloarthropathy is difficult to confirm in childhood and may become more obvious in the early adult years. A dramatic response to antiinflammatory medication may raise the level of suspicion. A premature diagnosis of a chronic problem can be upsetting to a young athlete and should be reserved for only those obvious and documented cases.

Those who have refractory pain that interferes with performance (and that persists after a reasonable work-up) often have to give up that particular sport. It is always difficult to make this recommendation to a young athlete. However, one of the mistakes physicians caring for spinally injured young athletes make is not restricting the patients long enough during their acute symptoms to prevent chronic changes and long-term sequelae. With the advent of all the diagnostic tests available, and the increasing expertise of physicians in the area of the child's spine, it is usually the exception where a diagnosis cannot be made and the young athletes cannot be returned to their sport following a spinal injury or problem.

REFERENCES

1. Bradford, D. S.   Scheuermann's kyphosis and roundback deformity. *J. Bone Joint Surg. [Am.]* 56:740, 1974.
2. Jackson, D. W., and Wiltse, L. L.   Low back pain in young athletes. *Physiol. Sports Med.* 2:53, 1974.
3. Jackson, D. W., Wiltse, L. L., and Cirincione, R. J.   Spondylolysis in the female gymnast. *Clin. Orthop.* 117:68, 1976.
4. Jackson, D. W., Wiltse, L. L., and Dingeman, R.   Sub-roentgenographic stress reactions of the posterior elements in young athletes. *Am. J. Sports Med.* 9:304, 1981.
5. Palmer, H.   Pain maps in the differential diagnosis of psychosomatic disorders, *Med. Press,* May 1960. P. 454.
6. Ransford, A. O., Cairns, D., and Mooney, V.   The pain drawing as an aid to psychologic evaluation of the patient with low back pain. *Spine* 1:127, 1976.
7. Scheuermann, H. W.   Kyfosis dorsalis juvenilis. *Ugeskr. Laeger.* 82:385, 1920.
8. Schmorl, G.   Die pathogenese der juvenilen kyphose. *Fortschr. Geb. Rontgenstr. Nuklearmed.* 41:359, 1930.
9. Sorensen, K. H.   *Scheuermann's Juvenile Kyphosis.* Copenhagen: Munksgaard, 1964.
10. Wiltse, L. L.   Spondylolisthesis in children. *Clin. Orthop.* 21:156, 1961.
11. Wiltse, L. L., and Jackson, D. W.   Treatment of spondylolisthesis and spondylolysis in children. *Clin. Orthop.* 117:92, 1976.
12. Wiltse, L. L., Widell, E. H., and Jackson, D. W.   Fatigue fracture: the basic lesion in isthmic spondylolisthesis. *J. Bone Joint Surg. [Am.]* 57:17, 1975.

7. Medical Problems of the Exercising Child: Asthma, Diabetes, and Epilepsy

Norman P. Spack

Asthma, diabetes, and epilepsy rank among the most common chronic medical problems that, despite their requirement for daily medication, permit the child and adolescent to participate in sports. In each condition, however, exercise has both positive and negative consequences. To maximize the positive effects, the physician must understand the influence of exercise on the physiology of the patient's illness. This will be discussed later in the chapter. First, however, we must focus on the impact of chronic illness on the psychological development of the child and adolescent athlete.

Early adolescents feel omnipotent, as their bodies soar into a growth spurt with concomitant surges in muscular development and strength. Rapid recovery from injury or transient illness confirms the adolescent's sense of invulnerability. In this context, chronic illness is a felt threat to the ego, and dependence on medications, special diets, and the attention of parents and doctors becomes interpreted as a sign of weakness. As adolescent patients deny that they are different from their peers (diabetics, asthmatics, and epileptics can readily hide their diagnoses), they will test the system, skipping doses of insulin, failing to use bronchodilators, or failing to take anticonvulsants until they are forced to admit that these agents are essential to prevent the more embarrassing consequences of ketoacidosis, status asthmaticus, or seizures. Maintaining a regimen is far easier for the older adolescent who has gained some mastery over his or her impulses and has the future orientation necessary to consider the consequences of an irrational act. Many will be guided by comedian Mel Brooks' description of mankind's greatest propulsive force: *"Fear!"* Fear of loss of control or, worse, loss of driving privileges, has kept many a diabetic eating the between-meals snack and many an epileptic on his medication.

Chronic illness poses a threat to the separation from parents essential for the psychological development into adulthood. Oriented both to the past and to the future, parents are intolerant of their adolescent's fixation on the present. Guilt over producing a child with medical problems may be overwhelming and, if the disease has a genetic basis, the parents will feel doubly responsible. Parents who are well feel remorseful for being so, especially when they are better adapted to handling a medical regimen than their adolescents. Overprotection is a common reaction to feelings of guilt and insecurity as parents attempt to shelter their child from the immediate and long-term consequences of illness. This intrusion, appropriate to the younger child, is often unacceptable to the adolescent who has an overriding need to establish his or her own identity. Nonetheless, adolescents may fall prey to some of the rewards of overprotection, and are ambivalent about the secondary gains of illness that may reduce expectation and excuse failure. At worst, the adolescent may feel a greater reward in being an invalid than in being forced to compete academically, socially, or athletically. Ideally, the patient-athlete will be in the care of a physician who supports his strivings for independence and plays the dual role of confidant to the patient and buffer between parent and child.

ASTHMA AND EXERCISE

Exercise remains a two-edged sword for the asthmatic child or adolescent. Whereas physical training increases the efficiency of breathing, exercise may precipitate or exacerbate bronchoconstriction. While changes in respiratory function are noted in the overwhelming majority of asthmatics shortly after they begin exercising, a smaller group experience bronchoconstriction *only* after an exercise stimulus. Exercise-induced asthma is, thus, one of the few pathophysiologic states affecting normal individuals in which exercise is etiologic.

Like their nonasthmatic peers, and in contrast to patients with chronic pulmonary disease with irreversible pulmonary function tests, asthmatics *increase* their ventilation during the first 5 to 10 minutes of exercise and maintain a normal arterial pO_2. Bronchodilation is noted during this interval, presumably due to the release of endogenous catecholamines [5]. Asthmatics frequently wheeze and/or cough after ten minutes of exercise, and are often maximally bronchoconstricted on return to rest, in contrast to nonasthmatics whose ventilation rapidly returns to pre-exercise levels when they stop exercising. Exercise-triggered wheezing or cough is accompanied by the typical changes of bronchoconstriction measured by pulmonary function tests: decreased forced expiratory volumes (FEV_1) and peak expiratory flow rates (PEFR) [8] (Figure 7-1). Hyperinflation of the chest reflects the increased functional residual capacity (FRC) and residual volume. Tests of their resistance and specific conductance indicate that both large and small airways are narrowed, with effects ranging from mild cough or dyspnea to severe bronchospasm and hypoxia. Severity of the attack is dependent on multiple factors including the pre-exercise pulmonary function. Spontaneous recovery occurs 30 to 90 minutes later.

Temperature and humidity of the inspired air are now known to be key variables in the etiology of the above syndrome [1, 12]. In the face of the increased ventilation necessary to maintain peripheral oxygenation under the exercise demands, the rapidly inspired air bypasses the normal intranasal mechanisms for warming and humidification. McFadden [12] has attributed the temperature drop in the intrathoracic airways as a critical stimulus for bronchoconstriction, an

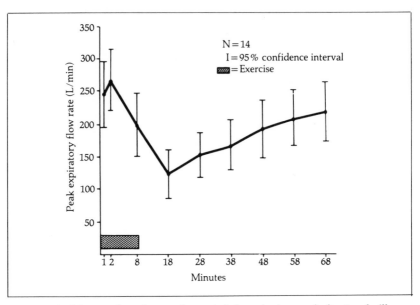

Figure 7-1. Mean peak expiratory flow rate before, during, and after treadmill exercise (walking 3 mph, 10-degree grade) in 14 asthmatic children. (From R. M. Sly, Exercise and the asthmatic child. Pediatr. Digest 14:42, 1972. With permission.)

effect proportional to the coldness and dryness of the inspired air. Air fully saturated with water and at body temperature fails to provoke bronchoconstriction regardless of the minute ventilation or amount of physical effort expended. In less optimal environments, when temperature and humidity are kept constant, the degree of bronchoconstriction is proportional to the minute ventilation. How intrathoracic cold air initiates bronchoconstriction is not known. The fact that some patients develop tolerance to exercise-induced bronchospasm after repetitive, brief exercise suggests that an offending effector substance may accumulate and deplete. Vagal mechanisms have also been implicated. Since cromolyn sodium, a drug that stabilizes mast cell membranes, has been shown to prevent such bronchoconstriction, the actual mediator substance may be contained within these mast cells [15].

Therapy for the exercising asthmatic begins with the recognition of the above factors by patients, parents, coaches, and physicians. Cough is not usually perceived as a sign of bronchial irritation or constriction, and coaches who ignore coughing or associate episodic dyspnea with an inadequte training regimen may mistakenly impose additional exercise and create a vicious cycle by which exercise induces more asthma [11]. Physicians must review the post-effort status of the athlete who may always appear well and free of wheezing at office visits.

Attempts to reproduce the wheezing in an office at 68° to 72° Fahrenheit are often ineffectual. Ultimately, the athlete must be in tune with himself, even avoiding prolonged effort on days when the internal (baseline pulmonary status) and external (temperature and humidity) environments generate increased discomfort. Maintenance of optimal pre-exercise pulmonary function via the usual modalities of environmental control and bronchodilators and the addition of specific bronchodilators taken before exercise provide the best hope for reducing dyspnea from exercise. The International Olympic Committee has listed cromolyn sodium and terbutaline sulfate as acceptable pre-event bronchodilators, in contrast to other beta-adrenergic agonists. The latter were well publicized when U. S. swimmer Rick DeMott was stripped of his Olympic medal after he had taken an ephedrine derivative for exercise-induced asthma, unaware that it was on the banned list.

Since the asthmatic athletes appear fine at the outset, they are not likely to be scratched from distance events by coaches or physicians. Many attempt to "run through" their asthma as they develop tolerance to the bronchoconstriction. Such a practice may be dangerous, for, as mentioned above, the symptoms may intensify even as the exhausted performer is forced to rest.

Selection of an appropriate sport may be the best prevention. Outdoor exercise requiring sustained ventilation (more than 6–10 minutes), particularly in cold, dry climates, presents the greatest problem. Distance running, cross-country skiing, and soccer are less well tolerated than activities requiring short bursts of activity with intermittent rests, such as dash events, baseball, and tennis. Because of the high environmental temperature and humidity, indoor swimming is probably the best tolerated sport.

Despite the above deleterious effects, exercise programs have been successfully used to improve the ventilatory status of chronic asthmatic children and adolescents. Sly et al. initiated a 13-week, 3-hour-per-week program for 26 chronically asthmatic 9- to 13-year-olds [16]. No specific changes in pulmonary function tests were noted at the conclusion of the program, although the exercising groups noted significant reduction in the number of days' wheezing when compared to a control group.

Similar results have been reported by other investigators in children with perennial wheezing: no significant change in pulmonary function tests, but patients improved psychologically and showed reduced severity of wheezing attacks and school absenteeism [7].

Rather than exercising patients through endurance training, these programs, which are taught by physical therapists, include breathing exercises designed to enable the patient to reduce hyperventilation by pursed-lip breathing and by voluntary contractions of abdominal muscles to improve diaphragmatic excursion and reduce air-trapping.

Physical training, specific breathing exercises, and selection of a sport appropriate for the temperature and humidity can reduce the impact of asthma on the athlete. Supervised experimentation with a variety of bronchodilators may be required to attain the best pre-exercise pulmonary function and the best athletic performance.

DIABETES AND EXERCISE

Salutary effects of exercise in the diabetic state were noted as early as the time of Christ by the Roman physician Celsus. The late Elliot Joslin considered exercise to be a cornerstone of treatment along with diet and insulin reconstitution (Figure 7-2). The latter is emphasized in the case of children and adolescents with diabetes, almost all of whom have the insulin-dependent (Type 1) variety. While these patients may retain some residual insulin secretory capacity, most have little or no beta cell response within a few years after diagnosis.

Instead of using a short half-life carefully regulated insulin release tailored to and responding to the blood glucose concentrations and suppressible by exercise-provoked catecholamines, insulin-dependent patients must control their metabolic abnormality with a quite different chemical. Proprietary insulins, derived from beef and pork pancreases,

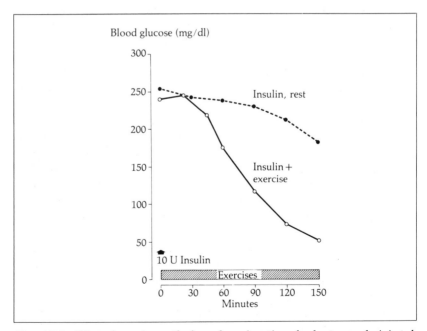

Figure 7-2. *Effect of exercise on the hypoglycemic action of subcutaneously injected regular insulin in a young man with diabetes mellitus of one-year duration. (From R. D. Lawrence, Br. Med. J. 1:648, 1926. With permission.)*

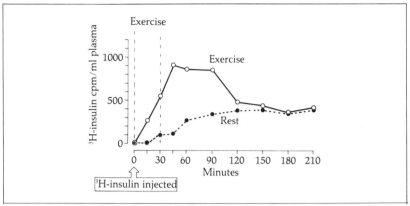

Figure 7-3. Effect of mild bicycle exercise on plasma levels of intact [³H] insulin following subcutaneous injection of 4 × 10⁵ cpm [³H] insulin/kg body weight into the leg of a juvenile diabetic patient (without circulating insulin antibodies). (From M. Vranic and M. Berger, Exercise and diabetes mellitus. Diabetes 28 [Supp. 1]: 147, 1975. With permission.)

differ in amino acid structure from human insulin and produce an idiosyncratic antibody response in the recipient that alters the functional half-life of the injected insulin. Once administered into the subcutaneous fat, insulin is absorbed directly into the systemic circulation instead of the portal vein that normally "insulizes" the liver before reaching the peripheral tissues. Variables such as the site of injection (amount of induration), depth and technique of injection, and rate of blood flow through the site determine the rate of absorption. Exercising limbs pick up subcutaneous insulin at a faster rate, despite the diminished insulin requirements of the exercising patient [9] (Figure 7-3). Physiologic factors that suppress insulin release from the normal beta cell are inoperative when the insulin is released from fat depots. In short, insulin therapy forces the patient's brain to substitute for the beta cell as computer, integrating all variables that influence glycemia and altering the therapeutic triad (exercise, insulin, and diet) to maintain metabolic balance.

Fortunately, microvascular (retinopathic and nephropathic), macrovascular (angiopathic), and neuropathic complications are rarely evident in children and adolescents with diabetes and do not compromise their athletic participation. Diabetics do have an increased tendency towards hypercholesterolemia and earlier coronary vascular disease, however. The type of pattern characterizing their hyperlipidemia has been shown by Sosenko et al. to correlate with degree of glycemic control as measured by such long-term integrators as glycosylated hemoglobin (hemoglobin A_1) measurements [17]. Physical training has been associated with an increased fraction of the high

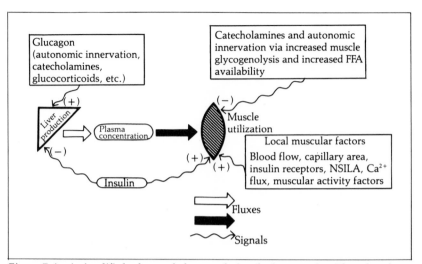

Figure 7-4. A simplified scheme of glucoregulation during exercise. The roles of insulin and glucagon are emphasized. (From M. Vranic and M. Berger, Exercise and diabetes mellitus. Diabetes 28 *[Supp. 1]: 147, 1975. With permission.)*

density lipoprotein (HDL) cholesterol that appears to have a protective effect on the risk for coronary vascular disease [4]. All the above benefits notwithstanding, exercise presents special problems for diabetics in terms of precipitating hyperglycemia with ketosis or hypoglycemia with its confusional states and seizures.

While resting skeletal muscle is fueled almost exclusively by fatty acids, exercising muscles also burn carbohydrates [3]. By mechanisms not wholly understood, glucose uptake is enhanced in exercising muscles. The various factors which affect glucoregulation during exercise are summarized in Figure 7-4 and the following points should be emphasized [18]:

1. Insulin plays a key role in the glucose uptake of exercising muscles, possibly via increased binding of insulin to its receptors.
2. Insulin also blocks hepatic glucose production via suppression of glycogenolysis.
3. Catecholamines suppress beta cell release of insulin.
4. Catecholamines can also increase the availability of muscle fuels via mobilization of free fatty acids (FFA) from fat cells and by promoting muscle glycogenolysis.
5. When relative or absolute insulin deficiency prevents glucose uptake by muscle, the concentration of glucose in the peripheral blood can be expected to rise.

Whereas well-controlled diabetics may respond to exercise with hypoglycemia via increased net uptake of glucose by the muscle and diminished glucose output by the liver, poorly controlled patients may exhibit a *hyper*glycemic response, often with ketosis. Ketotic diabetics have been shown to have an exaggerated catecholamine response to exercise, which may be triggered by the exercise-induced initial fall in blood glucose concentration [2]. Physical training results in two factors that reduce the likelihood of a deleterious blood-glucose response to exercise. First, fatty acids rather than carbohydrates become the preferred fuel for the muscle. Secondly, the catecholamine response to exercise is reduced in trained subjects, thereby diminishing the tendency towards ketosis [6].

Since fatty acids are incapable of providing *all* muscle energy requirements in prolonged exercise such as distance running, carbohydrates must provide the remaining energy supply. Since carbohydrates are burned at a constant rate, hepatic glucose output is the only mechanism for maintaining the supply in the fasting exercising subject. Once the liver supply is exhausted, hypoglycemia supervenes. Even nondiabetics must refuel their livers with ingested carbohydrate during marathons lest they develop serious hypoglycemia [10]. It is, therefore, essential that exercising diabetics get into the best control possible so that they may derive the benefits and none of the risks of exercise. This will usually require more than one injection of insulin per day, often combining short- and intermediate-acting preparations before breakfast and supper. When glycosuria fails to provide a reliable index of control and when accurate blood glucose concentrations are sought, patients can obtain fingerstick readings using a Dextrostick with a reflectance meter or a Chemstrip-BG that can be read easily without any metering device. Prevention of insulin reactions requires availability of 10 to 15 grams of quick-acting carbohydrate, as may be provided by 2 to 4 Life-Savers. Distance runners and bikers must prophylactically consume carbohydrate throughout the event. Injections given on the day of vigorous activity are best given into the subcutaneous tissue of the abdomen. The increased absorption of insulin from the exercising leg increases the uptake of glucose by the muscles while suppressing hepatic glucose output. The resulting imbalance renders the patient especially vulnerable to hypoglycemia.

EPILEPSY AND EXERCISE

For patients with epilepsy, exercise appears to have predominately beneficial effects. Nevertheless, the epileptic shares the diabetic's risk for sudden changes in mental status. While many epileptics have been seizure-free as the result of anticonvulsant therapy, many "break through" consequent to a change of medication or dose, lack of compliance with medication, episodic illness, or ingestion of substances, such as alcohol, that lower the seizure threshold.

Unlike the diabetic who should be able to anticipate hypoglycemic coma (via the signals of hunger, diaphoresis, or tremor) and reverse the event via ingestion of rapidly absorbed carboyhydrate, the epileptic has little warning even if he senses an aura, and has little recourse for aborting the seizure. Consequently, epileptics should avoid sports such as high-diving, rock-climbing, hang-gliding, and spelunking where even a minor seizure could lead to disastrous consequences. This recommendation must be tempered by the knowledge that the *most* serious seizures, major motor spells, are least likely to occur during exercise when the adrenergic and reticular activating system stimulation suppresses the epileptiform discharges. Sleep and the "twilight zone" between sleep and wakefulness are more opportune times for both aberrant central nervous system electrical activity and clinical seizures. Although the risk of drowning has been shown to be extremely small in a study of Hawaiian and Australian epileptic children, the risk is increased compared to nonepileptics. Epilepsy was a contributing cause in 4 percent of the 300 consecutive cases of serious immersion accidents, but all fatal events attributable to epilepsy occurred in the bathtub [14]. Consequently, the 1980 *Year Book of Pediatrics* recommends that "an epileptic child may swim with confidence provided he has been free from seizures for a year, has an adequate blood anticonvulsant level, and is supervised in the water by an adult" [13].

The most positive effect of exercise for the epileptic may be the knowledge that he is least likely to be compromised by a seizure while exercising. The exercise itself fosters a sense of well-being by affirming that the epileptic is capable of performing and competing.

In conclusion, then, asthma is an episodic condition that often disappears with time. Both the epileptic and diabetic face the prospect that, although improved therapy may control their condition, they will always be dependent on some daily medical regimen. The diabetic approaches adulthood cognizant of the potential for micro- and macrovascular complications that affect both the quality and quantity of life. Asthmatics have rarely been stigmatized; epileptics remain so and are thus disinclined to advertise their condition. Diabetics, partly as the result of the public education efforts of national foundations and the testimonies of public personalities who have diabetes, have recently "come out of the closet." It is no small consolation to the adolescent diabetic athlete that professionals such as tennis players Ham Richardson and Bill Talbert, baseball's Ron Santo and Catfish Hunter, and hockey's Bobby Clarke have performed while balancing their diet, insulin, and exercise.

Not only have these athletes demonstrated that their medical condition need not be a constraint to a successful sports career, but their recent discussions of their medical regimens in such lay publications as *Diabetes Forecast* have reaffirmed a fundamental point shared by other diabetics as well as by asthmatics and epileptics: their exercise program not only adds to the overall quality of life but enhances their ability to control their medical problem.

REFERENCES

1. Bar-Or, O., Neuman, I., and Dotan, R. Effects of dry and humid climates on exercise-induced asthma in children and pre-adolescents. *J. Allergy Clin. Immunol.* 60:163, 1977.
2. Christensen, N. J., et al. Catecholamines and exercise. In M. Vranic, J. Wahren, and S. Hovarth (Eds.), Proceedings of Conference on Diabetes and Exercise. *Diabetes* 28 (Suppl. 1): 58, 1979.
3. Felig P., and Wahren, J. Fuel homeostasis in exercise. *N. Engl. J. Med.* 293:1078, 1975.
4. Garcia-Palmeri, M. R., et al. Interrelation of serum lipids with relative weight, blood glucose and physical activity. *Circulation* 45:829, 1972.
5. Griffiths, J., et al. Sequential examination of plasma catecholamines in exercised-induced asthma. *Chest* 62:527, 1972.
6. Hartley, L. H., et al. Multiple hormonal responses to graded exercise in relation to physical training. *J. Appl. Physiol.* 33:602, 1972.
7. Hyde, J. S., and Swarts, C. L. Effect of an exercise program on the perennially asthmatic child. *Am. J. Dis. Child.* 116:383, 1968.
8. Katz, R. M., et al. Exercised-induced bronchospasm, ventilation and blood gases in asthmatic children. *J. Allergy* 45:148, 1971.
9. Koivisto, V. A., and Felig, P. Effects of leg exercise on insulin absorption in diabetic patients. *N. Engl. J. Med.* 298:77, 1978.
10. Levine, S. A., Gordon, B., and Derick, C. L. Some changes in the chemical constituents of the blood following a marathon race. *J.A.M.A.* 82:1778, 1924.
11. McFadden, E. R. Exertional dyspnea and cough as preludes to acute attacks of bronchial asthma. *N. Engl. J. Med.* 292:555, 1975.
12. McFadden, E. R., and Ingram, R. H. Exercised-induced asthma. Observations on the initiating stimulus. *N. Engl. J. Med.* 301:763, 1979.
13. Oski, F. A., and Stockman, J. A. *Year Book of Pediatrics, 1980.* Chicago: Year Book, 1980.
14. Pearn, J., Bart, R., and Yamoaka, R. Drowning risks to epileptic children. *Br. Med. J.* 2:1248, 1978.
15. Poppius, H., et al. Exercise asthma and disodium cromoglycate. *Br. Med. J.* 4:337, 1970.
16. Sly, R. M., Harper, R. T., and Rosselot, I. The effect of physical conditioning upon asthmatic children. *Ann. Allergy* 30:86, 1972.
17. Sosenko, J. M., et al. Hyperglycemia and plasma lipid levels. *N. Engl. J. Med.* 302:650, 1980.
18. Vranic, M., and Berger, M. Exercise and diabetes mellitus. *Diabetes* 28 (Supp.1):147, 1975.

ADDITIONAL READING

Bierman, C. W., and Person, W. E. (Eds.). Symposium on exercise and asthma. *Pediatrics* 56:843, 1975.
Cropp, G. J. A. Exercise-induced asthma. *Pediatr. Clin. North Am.* 22:63, 1978.
Shephard, R. J. Exercise-induced bronchospasm—a review. *Med. Sci. Sports* 9:11, 1977.
Sly, R. M. Exercise-induced Asthma. In E. B. Weiss and M. A. Segal (Eds.), *Bronchial Asthma: Mechanisms and Therapeutics.* Boston: Little, Brown, 1976.

8. Nutrition in Children's Sports

Nathan J. Smith

Informed nutrition counseling of the young athlete can prevent abusive and potentially hazardous nutrition practices, optimize athletic performance, and introduce the athlete and his family to sound dietary practices that may have life-long benefits. The desire to succeed in sports can be a powerful motivation for good health practices among increasing numbers of young sport participants.

THE BASIC DIET AND AVOIDING SUPPLEMENTS

The young athlete should know that intense physical activity, training, and athletic competition do not inordinately increase the need for any specific nutrient. Exercise only greatly increases the need for energy and water. There is no increase in the requirement for protein, vitamins, minerals, amino acids, etc., that will not be met optimally through food intake that satisfies energy needs of the active young athlete [7]. There is likewise no nutrient that will enhance athletic performance when taken in larger than usual amounts. Thus, there is no place in the diet of the healthy athlete for the vitamin, protein, or mineral supplements that are so vigorously promoted to the highly motivated but uninformed and vulnerable population of athletes.

A diet pattern that will include a sufficient intake of all essential nutrients is referred to as the athlete's "basic diet" [8]. Such a diet makes protein and vitamin supplements unnecessary and wastefully expensive, as well as potentially dangerous. The athlete's basic diet need only be modified on special occasions to meet some very particular energy needs of different types of competition.

In counseling the young athlete regarding his basic diet, the physician may use the four- or five-food group plan most young people have been taught by the time they reach high school. The athlete can be assured that all of his or her needs for essential nutrients will be met with two servings of each of the dairy and high protein groups of foods and four servings each day from the grain and cereal group and four servings from the fruits and vegetables group. Depending on the foods selected, these 12 servings will provide only 1200 to 1500 kcal. However, this is an inadequate energy intake for any young athlete. Thus, the basic diet is one that insures a good intake of essential nutrients, but is a diet to which second helpings and preference foods are added to satisfy energy needs and to assure that a desired weight for competition is maintained. The active boy or girl is reminded to "first eat what you need (the basic diet), then eat what you want."

The basic diet based on the food groups will not satisfy the iron requirement of 10 percent to 15 percent of women athletes. The iron content of even a high-quality American diet is not great and, when coupled with the body's limited ability to absorb iron, requires that 1 in 8 to 10 normal women will need to regularly use a medicinal iron supplement during their years of menstrual iron loss.

THE BENEFITS OF REGULAR INTAKES OF ENERGY

The intake of energy periodically throughout the day as well as with daily regularity during a training period is essential in meeting the energy demands of the athlete. The well-nourished, large high-school boy will have at any one time no more than 1200 to 1400 kcal of readily available energy as carbohydrate stores in various body compartments. This energy can meet the demands of less than 12 hours of sedentary school day activities. The young person who frequently misses breakfast, and whose lunch is little more than an unpredictable snack, will come into an afternoon training session with inadequate energy to perform well. Regular meal-time eating three or more times a day is the surest way for the athlete to provide for the energy needs of training and competition. The all too popular eating pattern of one large evening meal and intermittent, irregular snacks during the day will often send the athlete into practice or competition seriously lacking in available energy stores.

Using analysis of serial muscle biopsies, Costill and his co-workers have demonstrated that too intense training and limited energy intakes preceding competition can deplete muscle glycogen reserves [2]. Compromising this important source of energy contributes to so-called staleness and underperformance. Distance runners training with daily long runs even while taking in a generous diet were shown to experience progressively lower concentrations of muscle glycogen each day. Reduced intensity in training for three or more days while continuing to take a good diet was needed to replenish the glycogen stores and to optimize muscle energy available for the day of competition. The message from these studies is the necessity for regular and continuing good food energy intakes during training and reducing the intensity of training several days before important games or meets. All high-energy-output athletes will perform better if they satisfy their demands for regular and continuing needs for energy. This includes the basketball player, the distance runner or swimmer, the soccer player, the cross-country skier, the player of racquet sports, etc.

OPTIMIZING ENERGY FOR DIFFERENT SPORTS

The serious boy or girl athlete will often benefit from informed advice as to how to best meet the specific energy needs of differing types of sports or competitions.

In certain athletic events of very short duration such as the 50-yard dash, the pole vault, or certain types of gymnastic competitions, the brief periods of competition are separated by significant rest periods. Essentially all of these sports demand that body fat be reduced to a healthy minimum. Diet and training schedules in the pre-season should be managed to achieve the desired level of fatness and a stable competing weight [9]. These short duration contests involve short outbursts of anaerobic energy supplied by adenosine triphosphate (ATP) and phosphocreatine. In preparing for competition of this nature, attention is given to a good dietary intake for several days preceding the contest, maintenance of a good level of hydration, and regular, planned high-carbohydrate intakes such as fruit juices or light meals.

Maintaining a good fluid intake is essential in all types of exercise and is often overlooked, particularly by girl athletes. In the intense environment of competition, thirst is no reliable indicator of fluid needs. Scheduled intake of water or very dilute fruit juice every 60 to 90 minutes is an effective way of providing for adequate hydration.

A diet that is adequate to meet energy needs and accompanied by generous intakes of cool, palatable water will satisfy the needs of maintenance of body fluids and will also meet the needs of electrolyte replacement. Thus, commercially available electrolyte beverages, and particularly salt tablets, are best avoided. Homemade electrolyte mixtures as well as many highly promoted products may be unpalatable and may interfere with adequate water intake. They are all unnecessary for the well-nourished and well-hydrated athlete. Clean, cool water is the ideal beverage for the athlete.

Contests that demand all-out efforts for periods of 3 to 10 minutes or longer, such as crew races, wrestling matches, middle-distance running and swimming races, involve a combination of both aerobic and anaerobic energy metabolism. These sports are among the most difficult types of events to train for. Muscle glycogen storage contributes significantly as a major source of energy in these types of competition [4, 6].

Performance is improved in endurance types of competition by a training and dietary program designed to maximize the glycogen content of muscles. This diet and training schedule is commonly referred to as "glycogen loading." Muscle glycogen stores are maximized by first depleting muscles of glycogen by restricting carbohydrate intake while following a vigorous training routine 6 to 4 days before a contest. Beginning 3 to 4 days before the event, the athlete eats a customary diet but supplements it with 1000 to 1500 kcal of low-residue carbohydrate foods or drinks. This provides the carbohydrate source to replenish and maximize muscle glycogen stores [8].

The diet and training schedule just described will produce maximal concentrations of glycogen in the specific muscle fibers involved in a given sporting event. A maximum amount of energy will be available to the athlete from this carbohydrate source. However, many young people will find the carbohydrate restriction that is recommended early in the week and the resulting depletion of muscle glycogen to have an adverse effect on their mid-week training performance. They are therefore choosing to avoid the low-carbohydrate intake during the sixth to fourth day prior to an important contest and program vigorous training early in the week, followed by high carbohydrate supplementation during the three days immediately preceding competition. The glycogen content of the muscle resulting from this practice will be slightly less than that resulting from glycogen depletion followed by carbohydrate supplementation, but is often less disturbing to the athlete's training schedule.

It is important to emphasize that glycogen loading is not a dietary and training routine to be practiced throughout a sport season. Glycogen loading is *only* recommended as a preparation by a serious athlete for an important competition of appropriate intensity or duration. It does optimally prepare the athlete for specific types of contests and if followed will assure the avoidance of ill-advised dietary abuses that can limit the athlete's performance. During the season a mixed diet adequate in energy containing generous amounts of carbohydrate will meet the daily training needs of the serious competitor.

WRESTLING: AN EXAMPLE OF
ACHIEVING DESIRED COMPETING WEIGHT

In many states the physician has been assigned by coaches and athletic associations the responsibility for certifying competing weight for the high-school and junior high-school wrestler. Parents will often seek physicians' advice regarding weight control by participants in wrestling programs. A well-planned weight control program should be provided for the aspiring young wrestler so that starvation, dehydration, drug doping, and a variety of other abuses can be avoided. At the present time as many as 200,000 American high-school boys may be suffering many months of growth arrest on markedly restricted diets during the wrestling season.

Several studies have documented a level of body fatness that represents an optimum ratio of muscle mass, strength, and endurance to body weight [11]. This optimal ratio will be reflected as the desired competing weight for athletes in a large number of sports as well as the desired competing weight for the young wrestler. How this level of body weight, i.e., body fatness, is achieved is of critical importance to the athlete.

Over the past several years a weight control program has been developed that can take the abuses out of high-school wrestling programs and at the same time contribute to the education, fitness, and competitiveness of the participant [9].

Soon after school starts in the fall the potential members of the wrestling team are weighed and an estimate of the level of fatness is made using a skin-fat-fold caliper.

It is important to recognize that the average white male high-school student from a middle- or upper-income family will have an excess of body fat. Recent population surveys indicate that a typical white, male adolescent living in an affluent family may have about 15 percent of his body weight as body fat [12]. Recent studies have demonstrated that 5 to 7 percent of body weight as body fat represents an optimal ratio of muscle strength, endurance, and quickness to body weight [11]. For a high-school boy with 15 percent of his body weight as body fat, a loss of 10 percent of body weight as body fat would be recommended. *Such a projected fat loss should occur no more rapidly than two pounds a week.* The wrestler's diet during this time would be a generous diet including all the basic food groups and providing no less than 1800 to 2000 kcal a day. This will be about 500 to 1000 kcal less than the athlete requires to maintain weight. Such a modestly restricted caloric intake still allows three meals a day, avoiding high calorie desserts and in-between meal eating. In addition to modest caloric restriction, fat loss is promoted by increasing energy expenditure by at least 500 to 700 kcal each day. This energy expenditure will involve an hour or more of running, interval training, weight lifting, etc., i.e., a general conditioning program that is prescribed by the coach [10]. Weight reduction induced in a teenage boy by increased energy expenditure and only moderate reduction in caloric intake will result in loss of body fat and will not decrease lean body mass. Severely restricted, "crash" diets will interfere with a normal growth and cause a significant proportion of the weight loss to be at the expense of the muscle mass.

It is absolutely essential that weight control through reduction of body fatness be started many weeks before the competing season. Weight assignments for competition should make allowances for growth, and the entire weight control program is best supervised by someone other than the head coach. A trainer, assistant coach, or team physician will usually be most effective in the weight surveillance of the young athletes.

It is important that specific steps be taken to inform parents, school administrators, school nurses, and community physicians of the basis and validity of the wrestling team's weight control program. Likewise, it is essential that weight and fatness be carefully monitored on a weekly basis throughout the competing season as there is a tendency for the reestablishment of once-established levels of over-fatness.

WEIGHT GAINING

There is appropriate concern about the widely publicized abuses associated with weight reduction and weight control in many sports such as wrestling, gymnastics, and figure skating. Less well recognized, but no less important, are the nutritional abuses of weight gaining or "bulking up" by a large number of young athletes, most often involving high-school and junior high-school-aged football players [5]. Without medical or nutritional guidelines hundreds of thousands of young men spend their spring and summer months attempting to gain 20 to 40 pounds of body weight on high-fat diets supplemented with a variety of useless and potentially dangerous vitamin, mineral, and protein supplements. This is nutritional abuse of the worst sort and is often compounded with the use of anabolic steroids and other drugs. These drugs are ineffective and dangerous, and their use is unethical [5]. They have no place in any athletic conditioning program.

American football is a popular sport. There are more than 1.5 million high-school boys participating each year, and large numbers of them desire to increase their body weight to increase their playing potential. These young men need nutrition counseling by an informed and understanding professional who can assess their growth potential as well as provide instruction for safe dietary practices and training routines.

In our experience a typical 16-year-old, 165-pound, six-foot-tall aspirant can gain 10 to 15 pounds of lean body mass and improve his potential as an athlete if he works hard, if he is highly motivated, and if he can afford the increased food intake needed to support this gain. The young athlete must recognize that if he is to increase only muscle mass and not become obese, only muscle work and not any specific food, vitamin, or hormone will produce an increase in muscle tissue. Experiencing a weight gain of 1 to 1½ pounds a week will require adding a modest-sized meal of 500 to 1000 kcal per day to his usual mixed diet. In addition he will participate in a program of muscle training for one hour several times each week. Each pound gain of lean body mass represents a positive caloric balance of approximately 3000 kcal. A weight gain of 1½ pounds per week is a maximum weight gain that one can anticipate if the weight gain is to be limited to lean body tissue.

Throughout the period of potential weight gain, skin-fat fold should be monitored weekly. An increase in skin-fat fold will call for an immediate modification of the diet and weight gaining program, increasing training, and decreasing caloric intake.

Large intakes of protein are to be avoided. They contribute nothing to a muscle gaining program and threaten the athlete with hyperuric acidemia and so-called weight-lifter's gout. An effort should be made to implement the necessary increase in caloric intake in weight gaining programs with fat-modified diets such as the American Heart Association's Prudent Diet for American Males. This diet reduces the saturated fat and cholesterol intake by limiting fat meats and dairy products, and can be a contribution to the nutritional education of every young man and his family. It is the only diet plan appropriate for increasing the caloric intake of the young athlete during a planned weight gaining experience. If the athlete's family has a history of early cardiovascular disease, the family is referred for blood lipid studies and appropriate follow-up.

IRON DEFICIENCY IN THE ATHLETE

Iron deficiency has been demonstrated to be a common problem in all recent nutrition surveys in the United States [12]. There is increasing evidence of significant limitations in both muscle work and central nervous system function associated with iron deficiency and iron depletion unrelated to the presence or absence of anemia [3].

In any population of athletes it is important to identify the athlete who may be suffering from iron depletion or iron deficiency. This becomes increasingly important as large numbers of girls and young women begin to participate in sports programs. Identifying the individual with frank anemia due to longstanding iron deficiency is rarely a problem in sports programs. The anemic individual is usually compromised to an extent not compatible with participation in high energy-expending sports. However, mild degrees of iron deficiency are common and may significantly limit performance.

Several populations are at risk of iron lack. The largest group comprises women who may become iron depleted after the menarche [1]. In studies of a large Washington state population there was very little difference in the frequency of iron deficiency among teenage girls in either low- or high-income families. Ten to fifteen percent are found to have degrees of iron depletion detectable by biochemical tests such as transferrin saturation, plasma ferritin levels, or erythrocyte protoporphyrin concentrations. Less than half of these girls will have detectable anemia. Iron deficiency in males in sports programs is limited to adolescent boys who are experiencing their rapid adolescent growth on irregular and inadequate diets. These boys are most often from poverty families.

Recent experimental evidence suggests that mild degrees of iron deficiency, as recognized by biochemical assessment using protoporphyrin or ferritin measures, may be associated with limited ability to perform physical work, i.e., athletic ability. The relatively low iron content of even a high-quality American diet, the human's limited ability to absorb dietary iron, and the rapid growth of present-day youth in affluent societies combine to place many at risk of iron deficiency. The possibility that iron deficiency may compromise the performance and motivation of the athlete makes biochemical assessment of iron nutritional status a rewarding part of the preparticipation health examination of all female athletes and of adolescent boys coming from backgrounds where their dietary intakes may be compromised.

THE PREGAME MEAL

It is important to inform the athletes competing in demanding endurance contests that Saturday's match is played on Wednesday through Friday's food intake. The pregame meal should not be looked to as the energy source to meet the needs of a high energy-demanding contest. The following guidelines should be considered in planning the pregame meal:

1. It should be planned well in advance of game day
2. The meal should be compatible with the optimal emotional preparation for the contest, taking advantage of the psychosocial aspects of food and eating to enhance communication among coaches and team members.
3. The menu should include any food that the player may feel will help his performance.
4. The meal should be low in fat, as fatty meals pass out of the stomach slowly.
5. The meal should be sufficient in amount so that the athlete is not hungry during the contest.
6. A modest contribution to energy needs can be provided with light, high carbohydrate foods.
7. The foods that have an obvious high risk of transmitting food poisoning should be avoided (turkey, gravies, cream pastries, etc.).

The traditional pregame steak meal, because of its size and fat content, leaves the stomach slowly. It has to be eaten 5 to 6 hours before a contest and many players will experience hunger during the competition. A simple, more appropriate menu includes fruit juices or a fruit punch, chicken and lean beef sandwiches, gelatin salad, sherbert, and cookies. This high carbohydrate, low fat meal can be taken 2½ to 3 hours before a game and may, with minor modifications, be boxed or brown-bagged from home by the low-budget athletic team. This simple menu can also be prepared at home by the young athlete when no parent is available in late afternoon to be responsible for the preparation of the pregame meal for a game at home.

Complete liquid meals such as Ensure Plus, originally developed for hospital use, are finding increasing favor as light, acceptable pregame meals. Such a beverage can be sipped in small amounts to within an hour or two before competition. For those athletes who direct their pregame anxieties to their gastrointestinal tract, the complete liquid meal will help avoid pregame vomiting, as well as provide some fluid intake and eliminate hunger sensations. These products may be used by some athletes as their only source of nutrition during day-long competition.

Tea and honey is a unique beverage combination that has considerable attraction to many young athletes. For the young participant who is not accustomed to caffeine drinks, caffeine intolerance can be experienced following a few cups of strong tea. Experiencing "caffeine jitters" is best avoided in preparing for a contest. Large intakes of honey will leave the stomach slowly and may create disastrous osmotic relationships in the upper gastrointestinal tract causing considerable distress and discomfort. Moderation is essential with all pregame food intake.

THE UNDERFED ATHLETE

The team physician and the coach should be alert to the nutritional status of the young athlete coming from a home in which there is insufficient food to meet the high food needs of an active young adolescent. Although an athletic experience for the young boy or girl from a poverty family may be tragically overemphasized in some instances, it can enhance self-image, be a tangible experience with winning, and be an important avenue to post-high-school education.

Nutrition surveys have repeatedly documented that the families in poverty buy food of nutritional quality similar to that of middle- and upper-income families, but for economic reasons the poverty family has less food [5]. When food is limited in amount, the individual with the greatest need is the individual at greatest risk of an inadequate intake. No one has a greater need for food than an active, growing, teen-aged athlete who is trying to participate in a high-energy expending sport such as basketball or soccer.

The adolescent male athlete in the poverty family is at particular risk as his adolescent growth is associated with a large acquisition of nutritionally demanding lean body mass. He may be iron deficient, but even more frequently he will be found to have an unpredictable and inadequate energy intake. Assuring an adequate dietary intake may have a significant impact on both the athletic and academic performance of the young boy or girl from the poverty family.

The young athletes' interest in athletic competition can prompt a high level of health concern motivated by their interest in optimal performance. Often this interest will be centered in a concern for good nutrition. Taking advantage of athletic participation to introduce young patients and their families to sound nutritional practices may provide important lifelong health benefits.

REFERENCES

1. Cook, J. D., Finch, C. A., and Smith, N. J. Evaluation of the iron status of a population. *Blood* 48:499, 1976.
2. Costill, D. L. Nutrition Requirements for Endurance Athletes. In E. J. Burke (Ed.), *Toward an Understanding of Human Performance.* Ithaca, N.Y.: Movement Pub., 1977.
3. Dollman, P. R., Beutler, E., and Finch, C. A. Effects of iron deficiency exclusive of anaemia. *Br. J. Haematol.* 40:179, 1978.
4. Fox, E. L. *Sports Physiology.* Philadelphia: Saunders, 1979. (Chapter 1.)
5. Frasier, S. D. Androgens and athletes. *Am. J. Dis. Child.* 125:479, 1973.
6. Karlsson, J., and Saltin, B. Diet, muscle glycogen and endurance performance. *J. Appl. Physiol.* 31:203, 1971.
7. Mayer, J., and Bullen, B. Nutrition and athletic performance. *Physiol. Rev.* 40:369, 1960.
8. Smith, N. J. *Food for Sport.* Palo Alto, Calif.: Bull Pub., 1976.
9. Smith, N. J. Gaining and losing weight in athletics. *J.A.M.A.* 236:149, 1976.
10. Smith, N. J., et al. *A Handbook for the Young Athlete.* Palo Alto, Calif.: Bull Pub., 1979.
11. Tcheng, T., and Tipton, C. M. Iowa wrestling study. *Med. Sci. Sports* 5:1, 1973.
12. *Ten-State Nutritional Survey, 1968–1970.* DHEW Publication No. (HSM) 72-8132. Washington, D.C.: U.S. Government Printing Office, 1972.

9. Psychological Impact of Organized Sports on Children

Linda K. Vaughan

Anthropologists [61], sociologists, developmental psychologists [54], and physical educators have been interested in children's play for many years. Play is generally perceived as an important component of the socialization and developmental process of children with spontaneity, creativity, and informal structure forming some of its essential elements. One advantage of play is the absence of adult intervention, which allows children to set their own standards and create situations where everyone can share in the joy and satisfaction of participation. From this viewpoint, the rise of organized athletics has prompted considerable concern about its tendency to reduce play opportunities for children. Devereux states: "I will argue that 'Little Leaguism' is threatening to wipe out the spontaneous culture of free play and games among American children, and that it is therefore robbing our children not just of their childish fun but also of their most valuable learning experience" [18, p. 37].

Several investigators have concluded that children now discard games two to three years earlier than they did before the introduction of organized sport [50]. Another author noted that youngsters participating in Little League had little time for play owing to the demands of the athletic schedule [110]. Early specialization has also been cited as a matter of concern related to the impact of athletics on play [57]. Sutton-Smith and Rosenberg [99] noted a trend in which boys spent more time on fewer sports, and, as a result, this significantly reduced the range of physical activities in which they were involved.

Although athletics traditionally have been supported from within the educational system, there has been an increasing trend for sponsorship by outside agencies. Participation of youth in these programs has been extensive and there is every indication that this will continue. In 1978 competitive youth programs involved 20 million children between 6 and 16 years of age [69]. A comprehensive study of competitive athletics in the state of Michigan revealed that children became involved in these programs at an average age of 8 years and as early as 5 years [74]. From the above, one must ask why organized athletics are becoming such a predominant feature of our society. Certainly play and informal games require far less in terms of facilities, equipment, personnel, and organizational effort. The proliferation of athletic programs would seem to indicate that the competitive experience in sports is highly valued in our society.

From the psychological standpoint, many people believe that participation in athletics helps to develop desirable personality characteristics, and that competition fosters social adjustment and helps to build character in terms of sportsmanship, cooperation, and leadership. Sports are viewed as a means for youngsters to release hostile and aggressive feelings in a socially acceptable way, and thus to reduce the problem of juvenile delinquency. The belief that sports participation is conducive to developing self-esteem, learning to cope with stress, and acquiring skills and attitudes to ensure lifetime participation represents a positive sentiment toward the value of athletics. Such beliefs, opinions, or myths are frequently cited as justification for athletic programs.

Since this point of view is so clearly in evidence in American society, one must seriously consider the psychological impact of athletics on children. Is the experience beneficial, harmful, or both? Despite the wealth of commentary on this subject, very little is really known about the benefits or consequences of athletic competition. Recently, however, concentrated efforts have produced some empirical data with which one can begin to measure the effect of competitive athletics on children and adolescents. The results of these efforts are the subject of this chapter. First, the competitive experience is examined in terms of personality and character development, and this examination includes the topics of personality, sportsmanship, cooperation, and aggression. Secondly, we will focus on competitive stress as related to self-esteem, anxiety, and motivation. Finally, the issue of adult involvement is addressed with respect to the influence of the family and coach.

PERSONALITY

Two schools of thought generally prevail regarding personality and emotional development. One holds that physical activity contributes to the development of personality; the other that sport has no influence at all on personality. The tension between these two opposing views has generated considerable research and commentary on the topic of personality. Research efforts have focused on either understanding the relation between personality and physical performance, or on identifying personality factors that can be used to predict athletic success.

While most research studies on the relation between sports competition and personality have utilized college students, less extensive research on children and adolescents has been done. One popular approach has been to compare athletes or sport participants with nonathletes or nonparticipants. Differences between participants and nonparticipants were found in several studies using self-report, teacher, and peer ratings. Seymour [75] reported that Little League participants scored slightly higher on personality traits both before and after the season, and showed a significant increase in social acceptance ratings from their peers during the season. Similarly, boys in Little League showed greater academic achievement and motor ability, and were better adjusted socially and emotionally than non-participants [82]. Children who ranked high on motor proficiency were also described as more frequently well-adjusted in social and personal relationships than those who were ranked low. Based on teachers' ratings, they seemed to have "more wholesome and well-integrated personalities" [58]. Similar findings were reported in a study of adolescents [4].

In another area of research inquiry, a positive relationship between sports participation and intelligence, physical performance, and personality has been noted [24]. Ray [59] found athletes to be superior in mental ability (intelligence and academic average) to nonathletes. In his review of personality research, Cooper [9] noted the need to distinguish between academic achievement and intelligence. He found no differences between athletes and nonathletes in measures of intelligence, but he did find significant differences in academic achievement. He concluded that athletes have more of an achievement orientation than nonathletes.

In contrast to these findings, Magill and Ash [36] studied children in grades 1 through 5 and found no significant differences between participants and nonparticipants in academic achievement, self-concept, trait anxiety, and motor development. Other studies have also reported no significant differences between competitors and noncompetitors in terms of personality or social adjustment [15, 44, 104]. And in a comparative study, Slusher observed that high-school athletes scored lower in intelligence [84].

One of the criticisms of the reseach on this issue frequently cited is that most of it has been one-time or cross-sectional in nature so that it is difficult to generalize findings beyond the sample involved. Very little longitudinal research has been conducted. However, two studies of this type examined slightly different variables and indicated that there may be an age factor to consider. In a four-year longitudinal study of elementary school children using factor analyses, Brown [7] reported that physical performance and emotional development factors tapped by a personality scale were discrete and not highly related. In another longitudinal study, athletes and nonathletes were tested over a three-year period. While the focus was more on sociopsychological factors, the results suggested that athletes possessed a higher sense of personal worth and self-acceptance than nonathletes. It was also found that the athletes had remained relatively stable while the nonathletes had changed appreciably since the initial differences between the two groups as measured by the California Personality Inventory increased significantly over time. The author suggested that this might be indicative of different rates of sociopsychological maturation [71].

Based on the belief that personality is an important factor in athletic success, many studies have been conducted to identify specific personality traits associated with selected sports, and ultimately to predict athletic success. In these studies college-age athletes, Olympic class performers, and professionals have been the primary focus, although some studies have been done on high-school and junior high-school athletes as well. The most frequent approaches have been to compare athletes with nonathletes, participants in team sports with those in individual sports, or to examine broad samples of athletes in specific sports.

Despite the diversity of findings, some supporting and some challenging the trait theory approach to the study of personality, specific characteristics are frequently used to describe the personality traits of athletes. Based on research on adolescents, these are dominance, tough-mindedness, extroversion, aggression, emotional stability, higher social acceptance, and high achievement needs [9, 18]. In contrast to the idea that the athletic experience shapes personality, it has been suggested by some sport psychologists that there is a gravitational principle involved whereby individuals with certain personality characteristics tend to be attracted to sport. In other words, athletes and nonathletes differ before participation, and there is a self-selection process that occurs [46, 80]. However, in order to determine if sport actually contributes to personality development or only attracts individuals because of their personality, longitudinal research will need to be conducted.

Many researchers have criticized personality research for its poor quality and confusing results. They point to sampling errors, poor methodology, inappropriate design, atheoretical hypotheses, and poor analyses and interpretation of results [9, 26, 29]. These critics argue that, even though the assertion of differences between athletes and nonathletes has some basis in fact, there is no evidence at this time that participation in physical activity and sports shapes personality [25]. Nor is there any support for the idea that athletes must have certain personality traits in order to be successful in athletics [29].

An opposing point of view to trait theory is the school of thought that supports a situational approach to the study of individual behavior. From this perspective personality is regarded as a nonsignificant factor in sport [63]. Based on the Skinnerian school of operant conditioning, several authors advocate that the focus of sport psychologists be shifted to areas such as behavior modification. They argue that prediction and control of sports behavior will be of far greater value to the study of sport than will predicting the athletic personality.

In this case the emphasis is on what the subject does and how to change that behavior by means of manipulating the environment, rather than on what the subject says or thinks as measured by self-report inventories [14, 62, 63].

Perhaps a more relevant, but infrequently addressed, concern is a recognition of the role of maturation in any study of children and adolescents. Most of the youth involved in organized athletics are in a period of rapid emotional, social, and physical development. If personality is formed in childhood and is modified throughout adolescence and early adulthood, then the impact of organized athletics on personality development can be critical.

CHARACTER DEVELOPMENT

SPORTSMANSHIP

One of the most common beliefs about the value of sports is that athletics contributes to psychosocial development, encompassing such qualities as character, good citizenship, morality—and specific to sports, the attitude of sportsmanship. This particular belief served as a rationale for the development and funding of athletic programs for many years. In 1971, Ogilvie and Tutko [49] created a furor by suggesting that, based on their research, there was no support for the thesis that sport builds character and that it may even limit development. They contended that sport serves as a selection rather than modeling process, selecting out more sports effective children.

Psychology has paid considerable attention to moral development, but not in the sports context. The basic issue is how moral behavior is influenced through competitive athletics, or whether this is even possible. Thus far there has been very little research on the issue [8]. Several studies involving children and adolescents looked at attempts to teach sportsmanship, but the findings were not significant. However, in these cases the exposure may have been too brief for any measurable changes to have occurred [6, 43]. Another study comparing athletes and nonathletes at the junior and senior high-school levels, reported no differences in attitudes of sportsmanship between the two groups. In fact, the evidence supports a decreasing or diminishing attitude of the importance of fairness and sportsmanship with increasing age. As measured by self-report sportsmanship attitude scales, the emphasis seems to shift from fair play to the importance of success and winning [34, 103]. If attitudes of sportsmanship are not being developed in sport, or, worse, if competition erodes already developed attitudes of fair play, this poses a challenge to all those involved in the conduct of athletic programs. For fair play in competition is the philosophical glue that our children are taught holds our society and political institutions together.

COOPERATION AND COMPETITION

Another belief that pervades our culture is that sport competition helps children learn to cooperate with others. Instead of viewing competition and cooperation as bipolar opposites, as mutually exclusive, it has been pointed out that in the sport context, children need to learn to cooperate in order to compete. Research studies of cooperative and competitive behavior in children have been confined predominantly to games in the laboratory setting. As a result very little research has been conducted in a more naturalistic setting. One exception is a series of experiments on in-group formation and intergroup relations by Sherif and Sherif [78], the results of which raised some serious questions about the instrumental value of competition. In these experiments with young boys in a camp setting, it was found that the introduction of competitive activities, including sports where there was an emphasis on winning at the expense of others, actually increased rivalry and hostility between groups. It was concluded that "cooperation and solidarity within ingroups need not necessarily imply solidarity and cooperation between groups" [78, p. 307]. However, a frequently cited experiment, the so-called Robbers Cave experiment, went beyond previous studies of intergroup relations by replicating the Sherif's results and then introducing superordinate goals to establish cooperation between the groups [77]. The implication here seems to be that in order to reduce rivalry or hostility developing between groups, a concentrated, intervening effort must be made to encourage cooperation within the competitive framework.

There has been considerable concern expressed about the emphasis on competition and winning in this country, especially in organized competitive programs for children. It is argued that prolonged competition on a win-loss basis can exert its influence beyond the game and has a significant impact on the psychosocial development of youngsters [76]. It has been suggested that games that stress cooperation rather than competition should replace the competitive game structure currently in existence [98]. Preliminary research in this area indicates that cooperative behavior in the kindergarten classroom can be increased through implementation of a cooperative games program [52].

The long-range effect of the emphasis of competitive behavior on psychosocial development at an early age has yet to be determined. However, there are indications that competition can have a dysfunctional influence on behavior between groups. From a social learning standpoint, it would seem that these behaviors should be examined from a developmental perspective with close attention to the competitive sports environment.

AGGRESSION AND VIOLENCE

On the notion that aggression is instinctive human behavior, sport has been perceived as a sanctioned situation where youngsters can release their frustrations and aggressive tendencies. Based on this premise, and the belief that the sport environment encourages and reinforces conforming behavior, athletics are believed to reduce delinquency. There has been very little research on this, but in a study of school and court records of 585 boys, Schafer [70] reported a relationship between delinquency and athletic participation that suggests that involvement in athletics may serve as a deterrent to delinquency. He cautioned, however, that this may not be the result of the athletic experience, but may be due to the fact that youths who conform are more likely to be selected into the athletic program. Additional support for selectivity as a factor was reported in research by Snyder and Spreitzer [94].

Another hypothesis regarding aggression is that the frustration that can be associated with competition may promote the expression of aggression or hostility [3]. The more popularly held belief at the moment, though, is that aggression is a socially learned behavior [12, 39, 85]. Many people feel that aggression begets aggression so that the more acts of violence are sanctioned and reinforced, the more likely they are to occur again. In a study of a highly organized youth ice hockey league in Canada, Vaz [102] concluded that aggression is learned, normative, and popularly sanctioned behavior in the sport subculture of ice hockey. There is also the suggestion that there may be an additive effect of exposure to sport violence that occurs as a result of mass media exposure, especially television [31, 85]. Martens summed up his commentary on aggression by stating: "Thus the implications are clear. Persons who observe violence and are reinforced for violence when participating in sports are likely to continue violent behavior" [39, p. 126]. The manner in which aggressive behavior is handled by those involved with the conduct of organized athletics is therefore very important.

We turn now to some findings on the effect of sports participation and competitive stress on the psychology of the child.

SELF-ESTEEM

In his frequently cited book *The Antecedents of Self-Esteem*, Coopersmith [10], reporting on research conducted from 1959–1965, identified self-esteem as an important behavioral characteristic. He defined it as "the evaluation which the individual makes and customarily maintains with regard to himself; it expresses an attitude of approval or disapproval and indicates the extent to which the individual believes himself to be capable, significant, successful and worthy" [10, p. 5].

Self-esteem is believed to be a relatively stable trait measure, although it may be influenced by situations. The development of positive self-esteem is considered to be a desirable outcome of participation in competitive athletics. Comparisons of athletes with nonathletes have shown that athletes have higher self-esteem scores on self-report measures than nonathletes [27, 47]. There is also some suggestion that self-esteem itself may have an influence on children's expectancies or satisfaction. In a study of young female soccer players, Scanlan and Passar [68] found that participants with higher levels of self-esteem and greater ability had higher pregame expectancies for successful performance than players with lower esteem and ability. In a study on Little League baseball it was reported that children who were low in self-esteem tended to evaluate their teammates and their sports experience less positively than players high in esteem [87].

As mentioned previously in the discussion of personality, athletes appear to hold a special status with their peers by virtue of their skill or physical maturity [17, 22]. If this is true, then lack of athletic ability may have a negative impact on self-esteem. Tentative support for this was found in a study of men who in their youth had been labeled as nonathletic by other children or coaches. The subjects recalled that as a result they had experienced feelings of inferiority and inadequacy. They felt that the sense of failure and loss of social acceptance had had considerable impact on their self-esteem [98].

Based on Marten's model of competition [39, 40], Scanlan [67] has argued that social evaluation is a key component in the competitive process. She suggested that competitive athletics may create a situation that can be perceived as a threat to self-esteem due to the potential of evaluation by parents, peers, and coaches. In a study of organized youth soccer, low levels of self-esteem were identified as one of the interpersonal factors that contribute to pregame anxiety [69]. In an effort to study the effect of coaching behaviors on athletes, Smith, Smoll, and Curtis [88] implemented a preseason training program for a group of Little League coaches in which positive reinforcing behaviors were encouraged. The authors reported that children who played under trained coaches showed a significant increase in self-esteem. Unfortunately these gains were measured at the close of two successful seasons and therefore their validity is suspect.

There appear to be a number of mediating variables that may contribute to the global concept of self-esteem. Among these are such factors as peer relationships, coaching behaviors, and physical abilities. Sex differences have also been reported [55]. If it is assumed that the sport environment has the potential for making a positive contribution to the development of self-esteem, then further research is needed to determine ways in which self-esteem may be enhanced. Since there apparently are many factors involved, innovative and multifaceted techniques will be required to critically examine this topic.

ANXIETY

The competitive situation is potentially stressful for the participants, and there has been longstanding concern about the effect of such stress on children in organized athletics. However, only recently have there been concentrated research efforts to study stress in terms of anxiety and performance. Spielberger's [96] concepts of state and trait anxiety have generated considerable interest among sport psychologists because of the theoretical differentiation between traits, which are seen as relatively enduring characteristics, and states, which are viewed as more labile and transitory. He defines trait anxiety as a behavioral predisposition through which an individual perceives certain situations as threatening or nonthreatening and to which the individual responds with varying levels of state anxiety. State anxiety is described as an immediate emotional response to a situation perceived to be threatening. On the basis of this distinction it is expected that individuals who are high in trait anxiety will perceive more situations as threatening or will respond to threat with more intense arousal or state anxiety [39].

One of the problems that has seriously impaired research efforts in the sport context is the lack of appropriate instrumentation. In response to this, Martens developed a sports-specific test to measure competitive trait anxiety, in order to predict state anxiety in varying competitive situations. The sport competition anxiety test (SCAT) appears to be a reliable and valid measure of competitive trait anxiety [40].

In a study of pregame anxiety, Klavora [28] administered Spielberger's State-Trait Anxiety Inventory (STAI) to junior and senior high-school baseball and football players. Measures were taken prior to competitive games and practice sessions. He found that all subjects, both high and low trait-anxious, had significantly higher measures of state anxiety prior to a competitive event. In addition high trait-anxious players scored higher in state anxiety (A-state) measures than low A-trait anxiety (A-trait) across all experimental conditions. In an effort to identify sources of competitive stress, Scanlan and Passar [68, 69] found that the major determinants of pregame anxiety in sports are interpersonal factors such as competitive trait anxiety, basal state anxiety, self-esteem, and performance expectancies for the individual and the team.

Postgame anxiety appears to be associated with situation factors such as win/loss or the interaction of win/loss with the number of games [68, 69]. Other studies have shown that after a series of wins, postgame anxiety (or perceived threat) is significantly reduced while in the case of a series of losses there is a significant increase in state anxiety [2, 66]. In summarizing some of her findings in field research on young male soccer players, Scanlan stated that, compared to players

low in competitive trait anxiety, high in self-esteem, and high in performance expectancies, "individuals who were high competitive trait
anxious, low self-esteem, and had low performance expectancies, experienced higher state anxiety when facing a pending competition
. . ." [69, p. 107]. Similar findings were also reported for 10- to 12-
year-old female soccer participants [68].

Stress appears to evoke heightened responses of arousal that are
measured by anxiety inventories such as Spielberger's STAI or Marten's SCAT. Physiological measuring techniques, such as galvanic skin
response (GSR) and heart-rate telemetry, have also been used in research on this topic. Using heart rate telemetry on Little League players, Hanson [23] found that emotional stress at bat was severe but
short-lived, yet subjects reported that they did not get especially
nervous. This suggests the need for using a combination of self-report
and physiological measures in order to accurately assess state anxiety
[97]. In another study utilizing telemetry, Skubic and Hilgendorf [83]
found that anticipatory heart rate represented almost 59 percent of
the total adjustment of the heart to exercise; also high anticipatory
heart rates were accompanied by high exercise heart rates. In this case
the authors suggested that heart rate may not only give evidence of
an emotional state but represent a physiological adjustment to the
anticipated activity as well. In his study of the relationship between
arousal and performance, Lowe [32] utilized a multifaceted approach
by combining physiological measures (heart rate and respiration rate)
with behavioral observation techniques. He also included in his analysis the effects of other contributing variables such as criticality of
both the game and the situation. In comparison with high and low
levels of stress, Lowe found that batting performance was optimal
when stress was moderate.

One question that arises at this point is whether the stress experienced in sport is more severe than other forms of stress in other
situations. In measuring galvanic skin responses of boys in Little League and the same boys in physical education classes, GSR levels were
no higher in league games than in competition in physical education
classes [81]. In another study, state anxiety levels of young boys were
compared prior to three types of evaluation: required school activities
(academic test, competition in physical education class), nonrequired,
nonsport situations (band solo performance, band group competition),
and nonschool sports. It was found that children involved in the band
solo situation manifested significantly higher state anxiety levels than
children in sports or required school activities. In addition, children
in individual sports participation had significantly higher state anxiety
levels than those in team sport. It was suggested that the greater the
evaluative potential inherent in the activity, such as in the case of
performing alone, the greater the state anxiety. Since 82 percent of

the anxiety scores were in the lower half of the scale, the authors suggested that, at least in this case, despite elevated anxiety levels, pre-event anxiety in evaluative activities did not appear to be excessive or overly stressful [79].

The effects of sport on anxiety and of anxiety on athletic performance are beginning to be explored in a systematic manner. Martens has made a significant contribution to sport psychology through his efforts to develop a model of competition and a theory of competitive stress [39, 40]. His sport competition anxiety test appears to be useful as a predictor of state anxiety in competitive situations. Efforts such as these are invaluable to the future study of the competitive process in sport, and it is hoped that future research will lead to an increased understanding about individual differences, desirable levels of anxiety, and ways in which anxiety can be influenced.

Motivation

Some comments were made in this chapter regarding the evaluative potential of the sport situation. If the competitive experience is viewed as an evaluative situation, then the impact of the situational variables becomes important. For example, there has been concern about the influence of external rewards on intrinsic motivation, and about the effect of negative or positive reinforcement on performance.

The emphasis on winning and the use of rewards have been of concern with respect to their influence on intrinsic motivation. Many people believe that the development and enhancement of intrinsic motivation is important if the basic purpose of competition is to foster enthusiasm and to engender satisfaction, which in turn will increase motivation for continued participation. Children play games not because they are made to do so, but for their own pleasure and satisfaction. Assuming most children are initially involved in organized athletics for their own enjoyment, what effect do extrinsic rewards such as trophies, rankings, winning, etc. have on children's intrinsic motivation? Deci's theory of intrinsic motivation has generated some interesting research. He proposed that "when people receive extrinsic rewards for doing those intrinsic activities, their intrinsic motivation may be depressed, unchanged, or enhanced" [12, p. 393].

In other words, Deci posits that there may be a negative or positive impact depending upon the saliency of the reward. In the sports context, many believe that extrinsic rewards reduce intrinsic motivation and result in a loss of interest and eventual withdrawal from participation. Support for this has been shown in several studies. In two studies a target drawing activity was used with preschool children whose intrinsic interest was already in evidence. The three experimental conditions were expected reward, unexpected reward, and no reward. Results showed that children in the expected reward condition displayed less intrinsic interest in the target activity in a free-play situation. Also on a pre-post analysis their intrinsic motivation decreased from the baseline measure [30].

There is some suggestion of a developmental sequence whereby extrinsic rewards may have a positive influence at first but later may be perceived negatively. Support for this view has been shown in a study in which the use of reward was examined from a developmental perspective. It was found that younger children viewed rewards as an incentive, but at a later age, rewards were viewed as a bribe [100]. Similar findings were reported in a study in which reward and nonreward situations were compared [22]. Thus far the research evidence suggests that in the case where initial interest in an activity is high, external rewards tend to have a negative effect upon intrinsic motivation. However, under conditions where initial interest is low, the use of external rewards has been shown to be highly effective [40]. This suggests that the conditions under which extrinsic rewards are utilized need to be carefully considered.

Instead of basing rewards on the product or outcome, it has been suggested that the emphasis should be shifted to the process or quality of the performance [12]. In other words, in addition to intrinsic (having fun) and extrinsic (winning), consider playing well and fairly [95]. This is proposed as a more viable way to increase and maintain intrinsic motivation in the competitive sports environment [12, 19]. Preliminary support for this approach has been found in a study of children on a target task [100]. Yiannakis summed up his concern regarding the impact of extrinsic reward on intrinsic motivation when he said: "Children who fail to appreciate the process of playing for its own sake and for whom satisfaction means winning seldom compete beyond their high school or college years" [105, p. 179].

Another situational variable of interest is the use of positive and negative reinforcement. It has generally been felt that positive reinforcement is more desirable for enhancing learning. Most of the research, however, has been done in a laboratory setting utilizing verbal or motor learning tasks. In an effort to examine the interactional process between the player and coach in a competitive situation, Smith, Smoll, and Hunt [89] developed an observational inventory that can be used to record a profile in terms of coaching behaviors. Positive and negative reinforcing behaviors are distinguished by means of the scale. The authors believe that there is a gap between what the coaches say they are doing and what the players perceive they are doing. In a study of Little League athletes, athletes reported more favorable attraction to coaches who used positive reinforcement in the form of encouragement and technical instruction. In a study where coaches were trained to be more positive in their coaching behaviors, children who played under these coaches were found to have more positive attitudes toward the coach, their teammates, and the sport experience in general [88]. In terms of positive reinforcement there may be a need to differentiate between different types of positive rewards themselves. Rushall and Pettinger [64] studied the results of various reinforcements in a learning situation and found that age was a factor in the effectiveness of selected positive rewards. Children 12 years or younger were more responsive to candy and money as reinforcement than the coaches' attention or postings on the record board. Those age 13 and over were not significantly affected by any of the reinforcement conditions. The authors concluded that coaches must consider the saliency of the rewards and the possible satiation effect in the use of reinforcement conditions to increase motivation or enhance performance. It would appear that initial level of interest, saliency of the reward (i.e., value to the individual), the nature of the reinforcement, and maturational factors are representative of some of the variables that must be considered when studying the complex area of motivation.

Adult involvement in children's sports has become an increasingly important area of investigation. Family and coach both exert a strong influence on the child athlete.

FAMILY

Research indicates that parents are a significant influence as socializing agents in terms of children's participation in organized athletics [33, 35, 86]. Generally, parents are considered even more significant than siblings as socializing agents [21]. It is known that the family plays a more influential role in early years, and that as a youngster approaches adolescence, significant others such as peers, coaches, and teachers begin to assume a role of greater influence [16]. Some of the research findings describe the same-sex parent as more influential in encouraging participation, especially if they themselves were sports participants [5, 93]. The most frequently cited significant parent, however, is the father [21]. Generally, previous sports participation, interest in continuing physical activity, and interest in sports in general usually result in either parent, especially the father, encouraging and supporting a child's involvement in sport and organized athletics.

On early attitude surveys, parents have consistently shown more positive attitudes toward competitive athletics than teachers and administrators. This was reported in the case of attitudes toward competitive athletics at the elementary level and in high school [72]. Considering the proliferation of organized athletic programs now in existence and the number of children participating, parental attitudes appear to continue to be highly supportive. The reasons for encouraging their children to participate no doubt are diverse and complex, but an underlying belief in the positive values of competitive athletics would seem to be the primary factor.

Recently there has been increasing concern regarding the dysfunctional role parents play in the social development of young boys and girls in sport. Some view parents as intruding into the sport environment and, by so doing, imposing their values on children so that fun becomes secondary to winning. There is also concern about adult expectations and the negative impact of this on children's levels of aspiration. In organized youth programs outside the educational framework, adults are serving as volunteer coaches, helping organize programs, and officiating. Many educators and sport psychologists have voiced strong criticism of the extent to which parents have become involved and the ultimate impact this will have on children [37]. Sage [65] said that the intrusion of adults is robbing youngsters of the opportunity to develop self discipline and a sense of responsibility. Several individuals and organizations have proposed bills of rights for athletes in which comments are made regarding the right of youngsters to be a part of the decision-making process [101]. Tutko expressed his feelings when he said: "I'm concerned with how many good athletes have been scarred by injury or burned out psychologically by the time they were fifteen because they were unable to meet the insatiable needs of their parents, their coach, their fans . . ." [101, p. ix].

There are suggestions that youngsters are beginning to drop out of sports in increasing numbers because of the adult domination of athletics. It is claimed that overemphasis on competition and overorganization has detracted from the fun and spontaneity of involvement [51, 69]. If adults continue to play such a pervasive role in athletics, some scientists are suggesting a change in the emphasis on winning or losing to the degree of success or a satisfaction of participation [76]. Another way would be to return sports to children and allow for more informal organization with children actively involved in the development and conduct of the program.

COACHES

Coaches have been identified as a significant factor in the socialization of athletes [35, 47]. In a certain respect the quality of the competitive experience is highly contingent upon the ability of the coaches, many of whom are volunteers and are parents of children involved in organized sports programs. Who are these people who serve as coaches? In an effort to address that question 423 male and female volunteer coaches representing eight sports were surveyed by means of a youth sports questionnaire. The respondents were described as being 91 percent male, with an average age of 36 years. Sixty percent had no formal training, and as a group they tended to have had six years of coaching experience. Most had children and 62 percent were parents whose children had been or were involved in the program they coached.

Coaches were in moderate agreement regarding too much emphasis on winning and tended to be more favorable toward their own program than sports in general [20]. In an analysis of orientation and goals, the coaches reported that the primary goal for youth involvement was socialization. They viewed themselves as more highly task-oriented in terms of helping children develop skills than affiliation-oriented through which fun would be emphasized [42]. In describing coaches from the perspective of value orientation, there have been suggestions that, due to coaching behaviors, the sport environment is a conservative and highly structured situation in which behavioral deviance is not tolerated [60]. For this reason sport was viewed as a way to reduce or prevent delinquency in earlier years [70]. Snyder stated that coaches tend to represent a conservative value orientation which tends *not* to "stress intellectualism, tolerance of unconventional behavior, or social and political liberalism" [92, p. 81].

Despite attitudes and beliefs, there is often a considerable gap between what people believe they are doing (self-perception) and their actual behavior. Several authors have proposed a mediational model to examine coach-player relationships in terms of observed and perceived behaviors [91]. Based on the premise that the interaction of the coach and athlete is a highly significant process, an observation instrument has been developed to record overt coaching behaviors. The classification system includes reactive and spontaneous behaviors. By analyzing this and utilizing an interview technique to determine players' perceptions and attitudes, considerably greater variance between perceived and actual behavior can be accounted for [15]. The model was applied in a study of 51 male coaches and Little League baseball players between the ages of 8 and 15. It was found that players generally evaluated their team members and the sport more positively if they played for a coach who gave high levels of reinforcement and support. In terms of attraction or favorable attitude toward the coach, spontaneity and positive reinforcement on the part of the coach rather than win/loss record were positively related to the players' attitudes. Perceived punitive behavior in terms of punishment and punitive technical instruction were negatively associated with attraction to the coach. In addition the results also supported the hypothesis that there is a discrepancy between what the coach perceives he is doing and his observed behavior [89].

It has been assumed that an experienced or trained coach is more effective than an untrained coach. Hence many organizations tend to give preference to volunteer coaches who have had either formal training or competitive experience. There is some disturbing evidence, however, that coaches with formal training or experience tend to place more emphasis on winning and less on having fun. They appear to be a more self-centered, winning-is-everything type of coach compared to coaches without training [42]. Further evidence for this viewpoint was found in a study of minor league hockey coaches in Canada, in which case a personality measure (leadership motivation) was more significantly related to coaching effectiveness than experience. The author suggested that certification programs should give more attention to leadership theory and its application to coaching than training in techniques and strategy [11]. In the case where Little League baseball coaches were given specific training in coaching behavior and sensitized to the impact of their behavior on the athletes, there was a significant positive effect on the players' attitudes and attraction toward the coach, teammates, and the competitive experience. There was also some indication of increased levels of self-esteem for children who played under trained coaches compared to those who did not. Unfortunately the basis of measurement for self-esteem spanned two seasons rather than a pre-post measure for one season [88].

There appear to be problems associated both with experienced and inexperienced coaches. Martens [37] identified these problems as errors due to lack of training and emphasis on winning. Because of this there have been requests for formal training programs especially for volunteer coaches working in organized youth athletics. Specific attention needs to be given to the proper care and treatment of injuries, teaching of techniques and skills, conditioning, psychological considerations, motor development, and nutrition [37, 88]. Efforts appear to be underway to begin to implement programs such as this, and initial results indicate that training programs can be implemented which will have a positive influence on behaviors and attitudes [88, 90]. Perhaps this will be the beginning of a concentrated effort to ensure that coaches are better prepared for their role and more aware of the potential influence they have on athletes.

THE CHILD'S RIGHT TO PLAY

What are the consequences or benefits of organized athletics? Preliminary research efforts are beginning to provide useful information that will help us begin to understand these complex processes. Generally one sentiment which has been expressed frequently is that mere participation alone does not ensure any positive benefits. In other words, as Martens so succinctly stated, "youth sports are not inherently evil nor are they inherently good—they are what we make them" [38, p. 214].

While the short-term impact of any psychological consequences may not be as readily apparent as physical injuries, there may be acute and chronic effects of the competitive programs. Normal, healthy children are amazingly resilient, but at some point cumulative experiences will have a significant impact on a child. Interest in this topic has primarily eminated from sport sociology and sport psychology. There has been some interest from other disciplines, but in a special issue commemorating the Year of the Child published by the American Psychological Association, no mention was made of sports or athletics [56].

There is an urgent need for us to increase our efforts to find out what sport does and does not do, so that measures can be taken to correct or improve the existing situation. Interdisciplinary efforts would be one way to approach the problem. In recognition of the complexities of behavior in the competitive context, recent efforts have been made to move from the laboratory setting to the playing fields. Applied field research endeavors should be encouraged and expanded [37, 87]. Teachers, coaches, and parents need to become better informed and sensitive to the potential hazards and the benefits in sports. One way in which to accomplish this is to make a concentrated effort to communicate with these groups and share with them the concerns and research findings of the professionals who are actively involved in the examination of these programs. In particular, the parents who encourage their children to participate and often volunteer as coaches should be a primary target in terms of informational efforts [37]. Of all the people involved in organized athletics, the athletes themselves are the principal figures. There needs to be more consideration for the athlete in terms of how he or she feels and what he or she perceives. The child is the consumer, but there seems to be very little interest in communicating with children and adolescents.

Inquiry should be focused on the impact of organized athletics on children who voluntarily drop out from the program, or who are selected out by the coaches and consequently labeled as unathletic [45, 48, 53]. Above all, the most unanimous collective opinion from those concerned with the youth athletic experience is that fun should not be neglected. The increased emphasis on winning has overshadowed this intrinsic value to the point that many youngsters now regard athletics as serious business. In a study of youth soccer the authors commented on the fact that the amount of fun experienced appeared to be related to postgame state anxiety and satisfaction with performance. Players who had less fun also evidenced greater stress. This is one of the first references in a research study to a factor which is generally regarded as being one of the more important values in athletics for children [69]. With respect to the emphasis on winning, other suggestions include less adult intervention, deemphasizing competition, less organization of the children, and encouragement of noncompetitive sports [61].

In conclusion, the *Guidelines for Children's Sports* published by the American Alliance for Health, Physical Education, Recreation, and Dance proposes a list of children's rights. It seems appropriate to end this discussion with an enumeration of these rights. Children, it is urged, should have

The right to participate in sports;
The right to participate at a level commensurate with each child's maturity and ability;
The right to have qualified adult leadership;
The right to play as a child and not as an adult;
The right of children to share in leadership and decision making of their sport participation;
The right to participate in safe and healthy environments;
The right to proper preparation for participation in sports;
The right to an equal opportunity to strive for success;
The right to be treated with dignity; and
The right to have fun in sports.

REFERENCES

1. Antonelli, F. Aggression and sport. *J. Sports Med. Phys. Fitness* 9:125, 1969.
2. Barnett, M., Corbin, C., and Matthews, K. The Effect of Direct and Indirect Competition on Children's State Anxiety. In L. Gedvilas and M. Kneer (Eds.), *Proceedings of the NAPECW/NAPEAM National Conference, Denver, Colorado.* Chicago: University of Illinois Press, 1978. P. 263.
3. Berkowitz, L. Sports Competition and Aggression. In I. Williams and L. Wankel (Eds.), *Proceedings Fourth Canadian Psycho-Motor Learning and Sports Psychology Symposium,* University of Waterloo. Ottawa: Department of National Health and Welfare, 1972. P. 321.
4. Biddulph, L. Athletic achievement and the personal and social adjustment of high school boys. *Res. Q. Am. Assoc. Health Phys. Educ.* 25:1, 1954.
5. Bohren, J. The role of the family in the socialization of female intercollegiate athletes. University of Maryland Ph.D. Dissertation, 1977.
6. Bovyer, G. Children's concepts of sportsmanship in the fourth, fifth and sixth grades. *Res. Q. Am. Assoc. Health Phys. Educ.* 34:282, 1963.
7. Brown, R. The Relationship Between Physical Performance and Personality in Elementary School Children. In G. Kenyon (Ed.) *Contemporary Psychology of Sport.* Chicago: The Athletic Institute, 1970. P. 439.
8. Chissom, B. Moral Behavior of Children Participating in Competitive Sports. In R. Magill, M. Ash, and F. Smoll (Eds.), *Children in Sport: A Contemporary Anthology.* Champaign, Ill.: Human Kinetics Pub., 1978. P. 193.
9. Cooper. L. Athletics, activity and personality: A review of the literature. *Res. Q. Am. Assoc. Health Phys. Educ.* 40:17, 1969.
10. Coopersmith, S. *The Antecedents of Self-esteem.* San Francisco: W. H. Freeman, 1967.

11. Danielson, R. Leadership Motivation and Coaching Classification as Related to Success in Minor Hockey League. In R. Christina and D. Landers (Eds.), *Psychology of Motor Behavior and Sport*. Champaign, Ill.: Human Kinetics Pub., 1977. Vol. 2, P. 183.
12. Deci, E. Intrinsic Motivation: Theory and Application. In D. Landers and R. Christina (Eds.), *Psychology of Motor Behavior and Sport*. Champaign, Ill.: Human Kinetics Pub., 1977. Vol. 1., P. 388.
13. Devereus, E. Backyard Versus Little League Baseball: The Impoverishment of Children's Games. In D. Landers (Ed.) *Social Problems in Athletics*. Urbana, Ill: University of Illinois Press, 1976. P. 37.
14. Dickinson, J. *A Behavioral Analysis of Sport*. Princeton: Princeton Book Co., 1977.
15. Dickey, B. A. Little League baseball and its effect on social and personal adjustment. University of Arkansas Ph.D. Dissertation, 1966.
16. Felker, D. Relationship between self-concept, body build, and perception of father's interest in sports in boys. *Res. Q. Am. Assoc. Health Phys. Educ.* 39:513, 1968.
17. Felkner, D. W., and Kay, R. S. Self-concept, sports interests, sports participation and body type of seventh- and eighth-grade boys. *J. Psychol.* 78:223, 1971.
18. Fletcher, R., and Dowell, L. Selected personality characteristics of high school athletes and nonathletes. *J. Psychol.* 77:39, 1971.
19. Gerson, R. Intrinsic motivation: implications for children's athletics. *Motor Skills: Theory into Practice* 2:111, 1978.
20. Gould, D., and Martens, R. Attitude of volunteer coaches toward significant youth sport issues. *Res. Q. Am. Assoc. Health Phys. Educ.* 50:369, 1979.
21. Greendorfer, S., and Lewko, J. Role of family members in sport socialization of children. *Res. Q. Am. Assoc. Health Phys. Educ.* 49:146, 1978.
22. Halliwell, W. The Effect of Cognitive Development on Children's Perceptions of Intrinsically and Extrinsically Motivated Behavior. In D. Landers and R. Christina (Eds.), *Psychology of Motor Behavior and Sport*. Champaign, Ill.: Human Kinetics Pub., 1977, Vol. 1, P. 403.
23. Hanson, D. Cardiac response to participation in Little League baseball competition as determined by telemetry. *Res. Q. Am. Assoc. Health Phys. Educ.* 38:384, 1967.
24. Isnail, A. H., Kane, J., and Kirkendall, D. R. Relationships among intellectual and nonintellectual variables. *Res. Q. Am. Assoc. Health Phys. Educ.* 40:83, 1969.
25. Kane, J. Personality and Physical Abilities. In G. Kenyon (Ed.), *Contemporary Psychology of Sport*. Chicago: Athletic Institute, 1970. P. 131.
26. Kane, J. Personality Research: The Current Controversy and Implications for Sports Studies. In W. Straub (Ed.), *Sport Psychology: An Analysis of Athlete Behavior*. Ithaca, N. Y.: Mouvement Pub. 1978. P. 228.
27. Kay, R., Felker, D., and Varoz, R. Sports interests and abilties as contributors to self-concept in junior high school boys. *Res. Q. Am. Assoc. Health Phys. Educ.* 43:208, 1972.
28. Klavora, P. Emotional Arousal in Athletes: New Considerations. In J. Salmela (Ed.), *Mouvement—Proceedings of the Seventh Canadian Psycho-Motor, Learning and Sport Psychology Symposium*. Quebec City, 1975. P. 279.
29. Kroll, W. Current Strategies and Problems in Personality Assessment of Athletes. In L. Smith (Ed.), *Psychology of Motor Learning*. Chicago: Athletic Institute, 1970. P. 349.

30. Lepper, M. R., and Greene, D.   Turning play into work: Effects of adult surveillance and extrinsic rewards on children's intrinsic motivation. *J. Pers. Soc. Psychol.* 31:479, 1975.
31. Liebert, R., and Baron, R.   *Effects of Symbolic Modeling on Children's Interpersonal Aggression.* Washington, D.C.: ERIC Reports, 1971.
32. Lowe, R.   Stress, arousal and task performance of Little League baseball players. University of Illinois at Urbana–Champaign Ph.D. Dissertation, 1973.
33. Loy, J., McPherson, B., and Kenyon, G.   *Sports and Social Systems.* Reading, Mass.: Addison–Wesley, 1978.
34. McAfee, R.   Sportsmanship attitudes of sixth, seventh, and eighth grade boys. *Res. Q. Am. Assoc. Health Phys. Educ.* 26:120, 1955.
35. McPherson, B., Guppy, L., and McKay, J.   The Social Structure of the Game and Sport Milieu. In J. Albinson and G. Andrew (Eds.), *Child in Sport and Physical Activity.* Baltimore: University Park Press, 1977. P. 161.
36. Magill, R., and Ash, M.   Academic, psycho-social, and motor characteristics of participants and nonparticipants in children's sport. *Res. Q. Am. Assoc. Health Phys. Educ.* 50:230, 1979.
37. Martens, R.   *Joy and Sadness in Children's Sports.* Champaign, Ill.: Human Kinetics Pub. 1978.
38. Martens, R.   Kid Sports: A Den of Inquity or Land of Promise. In R. Magill, M. Ash, and F. Smoll (Eds.), *Children in Sports: A Contemporary Anthology.* Champaign, Ill.: Human Kinetics Pub., 1978. P. 20.
39. Martens, R.   *Social Psychology and Physical Activity.* New York: Harper & Row, 1975.
40. Martens, R.   *Sport Competition Anxiety Test.* Champaign, Ill.: Human Kinetics Pub., 1977.
41. Martens, R., et al.   Competitive Anxiety: Theory and Research. In J. Salmela (Ed.), *Mouvement-Proceedings of the Seventh Canadian Psycho-Motor, Learning and Sport Psychology Symposium.* Quebec City, 1975. P. 289.
42. Martens, R., and Gould, D.   Why Do Adults Volunteer to Coach Children's Sports. In G. Roberts and K. Newell (Eds.), *Psychology of Motor Behavior and Sport 1978.* Champaign, Ill.: Human Kinetics Pub., 1979. P. 79.
43. Massengale, J.   The effects of sportsmanship instruction on junior high school boys. University of New Mexico Ph.D. Dissertation, 1969.
44. Meyers, C., and Ohnmacht, F.   Needs of pupils in relation to athletic competition at the junior high school level. *Res. Q. Am. Assoc. Health Phys. Educ.* 34.521, 1963.
45. Morgan, W.   Psychological Consequences of Vigorous Physical Activity and Sport. In M. G. Scott (Ed.), *The Academy Papers No. 8.* Iowa City, Iowa: The American Academy of Physical Education, 1974, P. 15.
46. Morgan, W.   Selected psychological considerations in sport. *Res. Q. Am. Assoc. Health Phys. Educ.* 45:374, 1974.
47. Morris, A., Vaccaro, P., and Clarke, D.   Psychological characteristics of age—Group competitive swimmers. *Percept. Mot. Skills* 48:1265, 1979.
48. Murray, M.   Organized Sport for Children: Growth and Development. In L. Gedvilas and M. Kneer (Eds.), *Proceedings of the NAPECW/NAPEAM National Conference: Denver, Colorado.* Chicago: University of Illinois Press, 1978. P. 189.
49. Ogilvie, B., and Tutko, T.   Sports: If you want to build character, try something else. *Psychol. Today* 5:61, 1971.
50. Opie, I., and Opie, P.   *Children's Games in Street and Playground.* Oxford: Clarendon Press, 1969. P. 1.

51. Orlick, T., and Botterill, C.   *Every Kid Can Win*. Chicago: Nelson-Hall, 1975.
52. Orlick, T., McNally, J., and O'Hara, T.   Cooperative Games: Systematic Analysis and Cooperative Impact. In F. Smoll and R. Smith (Eds.), *Psychological Perspectives in Youth Sports*. Washington: Hemisphere Pub. 1978, P. 203.
53. Pease, D., Locke, L., and Burlingame, M.   Athletic exclusion: A complex phenomenon. *Quest XVI*: 42, 1971.
54. Piaget, J.   *Play, Dreams and Imitations in Childhood*. New York: Norton, 1962.
55. Pomerantz, S.   Sex differences in the relative importance of self-esteem, physical self-satisfaction, and identity in predicting adolescent satisfaction. *J. Youth Adoles.* 8:51, 1979.
56. Psychology and Children: Current Research and Practice. *Am. Psychol.* (special issue) Vol. 34, October 1979.
57. Rarick, L.   Competitive sports for young boys: Controversial issues. *Med. Sci. Sports* 1:181, 1969.
58. Rarick, L., and McKee, R.   A study of seventy third grade children exhibiting extreme levels of achievement on tests of motor proficiency. *Res. Q. Am. Assoc. Health Phys. Educ.* 20:142, 1949.
59. Ray, H.   Inter-relationships of physical and mental abilities and achievements of high school boys. *Res. Q. Am. Assoc. Health Phys. Educ.* 11:129, 1940.
60. Rehberg, R., and Cohen, M.   Political attitudes and participation in extracurricular activities. In D. Landers (Ed.), *Social Problems in Athletes*. Urbana, Ill.: University of Illinois Press, 1976. P. 201.
61. Roberts, J., and Sutton-Smith, B.   Child training and game involvement. *Ethnology* 1:166, 1962.
62. Rushall, B.   A direction for contemporary sport psychology. *Can. J. Appl. Sport Sci.* 1:13, 1976.
63. Rushall, B.   An Evaluation of the Relationship Between Personality and Physical Performance Categories. In G. Kenyon (Ed.), *Contemporary Psychology of Sport*. Chicago: Athletic Institute, 1970. P. 157.
64. Rushall, B., and Pettinger, J.   An evaluation of the effect of various reinforcers used as motivators in swimming. *Res. Q. Am. Assoc. Health Phys. Educ.* 40:540, 1969.
65. Sage, G.   Socialization and Sports. In G. Sage (Ed.), *Sport and American Society Selected Readings* (2nd ed.). Reading, Mass.: Addison-Wesley, 1974. P. 162.
66. Scanlan, T.   The effects of success—failure on the perception of threat in a competitive situation. *Res. Q. Am. Assoc. Health Phys. Educ.* 48:144, 1977.
67. Scanlan, T.   Social Evaluation: A Key Developmental Element in the Competition Process. In R. Magill, M. Ash, and F. Smoll (Eds.), *Children in Sport: A Contemporary Anthology*. Champaign, Ill: Human Kinetics Pub., 1978. P. 131.
68. Scanlan, T., and Passer, M.   Factors influencing the competitive peformance expectancies of young female athletes.   *J. Sports Psychol.* 1:212, 1979.
69. Scanlan, T., and Passer, M.   Factors related to competitive stress among male youth sports participants. *Med. Sci. Sports* 10:103, 1978.
70. Schafer, W.   Some Social Sources and Consequences of Interscholastic Athletics: The Case of Participation and Delinquency. In G. Kenyon (Ed.),

Aspects of Contemporary Sports Sociology. Chicago: Athletic Institute, 1969. P. 29.

71. Schendel, J.   The Psychological Characteristics of High School Athletes and Non-participants in Athletics. In G. Kenyon (Ed.), *Contemporary Psychology of Sport.* Chicago: Athletic Institute, 1970. P. 79.

72. Scott, P.   Attitudes toward athletic competition in elementary schools. *Res. Q. Am. Assoc. Health Phys. Educ.* 24:352, 1953.

73. Seefeldt, V., et al.   Scope of Youth Sports Programs in the State of Michigan. In F. Smoll and R. Smith (Eds.), *Psychological Perspectives of Youth Sports.* Washington: Hemisphere Pub., 1978. P. 17.

74. Seefeldt, V., and Haubenstricker, J.   Competitive athletics for children— the Michigan study. *J. Phys. Educ. Recr.* 49:38, 1978.

75. Seymour, E.   Comparative study of certain behavior characteristics of participant and non-participant boys in Little League baseball. *Res. Q. Am. Assoc. Health Phys. Educ.* 27:338, 1956.

76. Sherif, C.   The Social Context of Competition. In D. Landers (Ed.), *Social Problems in Athletics.* Urbana, Ill.: University of Illinois Press, 1976. P. 18.

77. Sherif, M. et al.   *Intergroup Conflict and Cooperation: The Robbers Cave Experiment.* Norman, Oklahoma: Univerity of Oklahoma Press, 1961.

78. Sherif, M., and Sherif, C.   *Groups in Harmony and Tension.* New York: Harper & Row, 1953.

79. Simon, J., and Martens, R.   Childrens anxiety in sports and nonsport evaluative activities. *J. Sport Psychol.* 1:160, 1979.

80. Singer, R.   Athletic participation: Cause or result of certain personality factors? *Phys. Educ.* 24:169, 1967.

81. Skubic, E.   Emotional responses of boys to Little League and Middle League competitive baseball. *Res. Q. Am. Assoc. Health Phys. Educ.* 26:342, 1955.

82. Skubic, E.   Studies of Little League and Middle League baseball. *Res. Q. Am. Assoc. Health Phys Educ.* 27:97, 1956.

83. Skubic, E., and Hilgendorf, J.   Anticipatory exercise and recovery heart rates of girls as affected by four running events. *J. Appl. Physiol.* 19:853, 1964.

84. Slusher, H.   Personality and intelligence characteristics of selected high school athletes and nonathletes. *Res. Q. Am. Assoc. Health Phys. Educ.* 35:539, 1964.

85. Smith, M.   Social Learning of Violence in Minor Hockey. In F. Smoll and R. Smith (Eds.), *Psychological Perspectives in Youth Sports.* Washington: Hemisphere Pub., 1978. P. 91.

86. Smith, R., Adams, D., and Cork, C.   Socializing attitudes toward sport. *J. Sports Med. Phys. Fitness* 16:66, 1976.

87. Smith, R., and Smoll. F.   Sport and the Child: Conceptual and Research Perspectives. In F. Smoll and R. Smith (Eds.), *Psychological Perspectives in Youth Sports.* Washington: Hemisphere Pub. 1978, P. 3.

88. Smith, R., Smoll, F., and Curtis, B.   Coach effectiveness training. A cognitive-behavioral approach to enhancing relationship skills in youth sports coaches. *J. Sport Psychol.* 1:59, 1979.

89. Smith, R., Smoll, F., and Hunt, E.   A system for the behavioral assessment of athletic coaches. *Res. Q. Am. Assoc. Health Phys. Educ.* 48:401, 1977.

90. Smoll, F., and Smith, R.   Techniques for improving self-awareness of youth sports coaches. *J. Phys. Educ. Recr.* 51:46, 1980.

91. Smoll, F., et al.   Toward a mediational model of coach-player relationship. *Res. Q. Am. Assoc. Health Phys. Educ.* 49:528, 1978.
92. Snyder, E.   Aspects of social and political values of high school coaches. *Int. Rev. Sport Soc.* 8:73, 1973.
93. Snyder, E., and Spreitzer, E.   Family influence and involvement in sports. *Res. Q. Am. Assoc. Health Phys. Educ.* 44:249, 1973.
94. Snyder, E., and Spreitzer, E.   Life-long involvement in sports as a leisure pursuit: Aspects of role construction. *Quest XXXI:* 57, 1979.
95. Snyder, E., and Spreitzer, E.   Orientations toward sport: intrinsic, normative, extrinsic. *J. Sports Psychol.* 1:170, 1979.
96. Spielberger, C.   Theory and Research on Anxiety. In C. Spielberger (Ed.), *Anxiety and Behavior.* New York: Academic, 1966. P. 3.
97. Spielberger, C.   Trait-state anxiety and motor behavior.   *J. Motor Behav.* 3:265, 1971.
98. Stein, P., and Hoffman, S.   Sports and male role strain. *J. Soc. Issues* 34:136, 1978.
99. Sutton-Smith, B., and Rosenberg, B.   Sixty years of historical change in the game preferences of American children. *J. Am. Folklore* 74:17, 1961.
100. Thomas, J., and Tennant, L. K.   Effects of Rewards on Changes in Children's Motivation for An Athletic Task. In F. Smoll and R. Smith (Eds.), *Psychological Perspectives in Youth Sports.* Washington: Hemisphere Pub., 1978, P. 123.
101. Tutko, T., and Burns, W.   *Winning is Everything and Other American Myths.* New York: Macmillan, 1976.
102. Vaz, E., and Thomas, D.   What price victory? An analysis of minor hockey league player's attitudes toward winning. *Int. Rev. Sport Soc.* 2:33, 1974.
103. Webb, H.   Professionalism of Attitudes Toward Playing Among Adolescents. In G. Kenyon (Ed.), *Aspects of Contemporary Sport Sociology.* Chicago: Athletic Institute, 1969. P. 161.
104. Wilson, P.   Relationship between motor achievement and selected personality factors of junior and senior high school boys. *Res. Q. Am. Assoc. Health Phys. Educ.* 40:841, 1969.
105. Yiannakis, A.   Formal and Informal Play Settings: A Discursive Analysis of Processes and Outcomes for Children. In L. Gedvilas and M. Kneer (Eds.) *Proceedings of NAPECW/NAPEAM Conference, Denver, Colorado.* Chicago: University of Illinois Press, 1978. P. 175.

10. The Young Female Athlete

Lyle J. Micheli and Lana LaChabrier

The past ten years have seen a dramatic increase in girls' sports, both in number of participants and in types of sports played. This increased participation has been noted in sports with a tradition of female participation, such as field hockey, basketball, gymnastics, tennis, and softball, and in sports traditionally played by males. These "new" girls' sports include soccer, ice hockey, baseball, rugby, and even football. In addition, the growing interest of all age groups in fitness and recreational sports is shared by young women. The female jogger and cyclist is a common sight on most city streets.

A number of identifiable social forces motivate this increased participation. Equal rights legislation, such as Title IX of the Federal Education Act, and specific state statutes, such as Chapter 622 in the Massachusetts General Laws, require equal access for males and females to educational facilities, including gyms and playing fields. School systems at the primary, secondary, and collegiate levels are now required to provide men and women equal access to sports. In 1975, more than 1.3 million girls participated in 27 interscholastic sports at the high-school level, a 59 percent increase from 1973 [14]. Female candidates are now participating in the rigorous physical and athletic activities of our military academies, and women are vying for athletic scholarships at universities. Athletic participation and achievement, a traditional source of enhanced self-esteem for the male, have been encouraged by leaders of the feminist movement. Finally, weight reduction programs have begun to put more emphasis on exercise, and cosmetic and beauty firms have begun to stress the healthy and athletic look. Popular teen-age magazines such as *Seventeen* or *Young Miss* feature articles on weight training, running, and a great variety of topics related to sports and fitness in almost every issue. As a result, exercise and sports for girls have become accepted and even fashionable. Whatever the motivation, the arrival of these new female athletes has presented the coach, sports equipment manufacturer, sports physiologist, and sports physician with a number of questions.

INJURIES: DIFFERENT TYPES, DIFFERENT RATES?

A frequent question from parents, coaches, and physicians dealing with female athletes is whether there are injuries for which females have a specific predisposition based on physiologic or anatomic differences between males and females. Also, are female athletes at higher risk of injury from certain sports or athletic training techniques—either as a result of true physiologic differences between males and females, or perhaps because of cultural factors that effect the nature and type of preparation given female athletes. The answers to these two related questions have implications for diagnostic accuracy in girls' sports injuries, of course, but perhaps more importantly, for the prevention of these injuries, through structuring of physical education curricula, design of athletic equipment, and the organization of athletic training programs for girls.

The answer to the first of these questions is reassuring. Women seem to have very much the same type of sports injuries as males, and sex-specific problems are few in number [31]. Breast injuries, long cited as a contraindication to women's participation in contact sports, are probably one of the rarest injuries seen in women's athletics. A survey of college sports revealed several reports of breast contusions but no serious injuries [16]. In our own experience, while following four women's rugby clubs for a period of three years, we have not seen one significant breast injury.

Providing breast protection has been a concern in some girls' sports, however, and soccer leagues have frequently altered the playing rules to allow girls to protect their chests from a kicked ball with crossed arms. Certain women's hockey leagues use special chest protectors. Recently, a number of different support brassieres for women have been developed [15]. These are specifically designed to prevent discomfort rather than to provide impact protection. A survey of female marathon runners revealed that as many seem to be comfortable without support as those who use some type of breast support device [29].

The important sexual organs of the female are relatively better protected from serious athletic injury than are those of the male, of course, and serious sports injury to uterus or ovaries is extremely rare.

The menstrual cycle appears to have no significant effect upon female sports participation or performance, and some studies have been shown that vigorous athletic participation has decreased the incidence of menstrual complaints [2, 7]. Alterations in the menstrual cycle are not infrequent in the highly trained female athlete, however, and may prove worrisome. This is most frequently seen in endurance athletes, such as distance runners, swimmers, or skiers, and has also been reported in gymnasts, ice skaters, and dancers [10, 11]. These menstrual abnormalities—irregular menstruation or secondary amenorrhea—seem to be the result of a combination of psychologic and physiologic stresses in these athletes.

Recent work has suggested that this oligomenorrhea of the young female athlete may be related, at least in part, to nutritional factors in their athletic training [10, 13]. Specifically, the overall percentage of body-weight as fat appears to be a key factor in the initiation and maintenance of the menstrual cycle. Work by several different investigators have suggested a threshold level of adipose tissue below which menstrual function will cease. The same hormonal response that is thought to trigger oligomenorrhea may also be related to the occurrence of anorexia nervosa in the young female adolescent population [30].

These findings do not discount the importance of psychological factors in the occurrence of this condition. While sports training and competition can often help to dissipate stress in the teenager, they may also become a source of heightened stress, particularly in the individual sports such as dance, gymnastics, or figure skating. A reassuring study in this regard was done at the United States Military Academy at West Point [2]. A careful assessment of the complete entering class of 1976, the first class having female members at West Point, noted that 73 percent were experiencing discontinued menstruation after two months of training at the academy. After six months however, only 41 percent were still reporting secondary amenorrhea. After nine months, the figure was down to 29 percent, and after 12 months, down to 20 percent. After 15 months, all but 7 percent had resumed regular menstrual cycles. Interestingly, after this initial period of irregularity, approximately 55 percent of these women reported what they regarded as a favorable change in their menses after entering the academy: lighter flow, lesser cramping and discomfort, and shorter duration flow.

Long-term studies of adolescent athletes with these menstrual complaints are lacking. However, studies of elite athletes who have had this complaint are reassuring. No permanent impairment of reproductive or sexual function was found in a survey of 107 of the women champions in the 1952 Olympic games in Helsinki, Finland [18]. In addition, a study by Erdelye suggested that former international caliber female atheletes experienced a greater number of complication free pregnancies and easier delivery than recorded for a normal and less physically active control group [12]. It would appear then, that there is little sound medical or scientific rationale for restricting the normal female from participating in vigorous noncontact sports, and many reasons to encourage such participation.

A somewhat different, but nonethless related, concern regards the apparent delay of sexual maturation in association with vigorous athletic training that has been seen in certain young gymnasts and female swimmers. While clinical experience suggests that this delay results in no long-term deleterious effects, much more work is needed in studying this phenomenon before it can be dismissed as a safe developmental variant.

In summary, while our clinical experience with the complaint of menstrual irregularities in the young female athlete is reassuring, it must never be taken lightly. In addition to routine evaluation for amenorrhea, nutritional assessment, including determination of percentage of total body fat, should be considered. Consideration should also be given to psychologic or psychiatric review if evidence of high stress or anxiety is present. Simple corrective measures including change of training diet or exploration of stress issues may not only help correct this complaint but also avert other problems.

The second area of concern, whether girls sustain a higher rate of injury than boys, is more complex. There has been a traditional concern that females were at greater risk of injury from sports and athletic training than males. Proponents of this view have cited observed physiologic differences between males and females, and male and female athletes; differences in the performance records of elite males and females; and certain comparative studies or rates of injuries in certain sports which showed a higher rate of injury among female participants [8, 14].

Studies that have carefully determined the rate of injury in female sports participation are rare, and comparative studies on the rates of girls' and boys' injuries in similar sports are even rarer. Albohm conducted a study in 1976 on female high-school athletes throughout the country, and based on responses to injury questionnaires, she concluded that the difference in injuries between men and women were due to differences in sports played, and not to structural or physiologic differences [1]. In 1976 a study by Haycock and Gillette also found that women athletes sustained much the same injuries as men, except that the possibility was raised that women might have more joint injuries, e.g., ankle injuries, and patellar injuries [17]. A study by Whiteside that compared men's and women's injuries in comparable sports suggested that although the pattern of women's injuries was similar to men's, women might have a higher injury rate to the ankle in such sports as basketball and volleyball, and a higher injury rate in general in basketball and gymnastics [31]. Another study by Sullivan et al., of injuries in youth soccer, found that the injury rate for girls was twice as great as for boys in this new sport [28]. In both of these studies, however, the types of injuries sustained by girls and boys were very similar.

There is no question that we encounter many of the same types of musculoskeletal injuries in the female and male athlete—including fractures, dislocations, and contusions. These injuries, usually resulting from significant trauma, have a similar mechanism of injury and are managed identically in both sexes.

There is another group of injuries, however, that results from recurrent microtrauma arising out of repeated impact, such as in running in football or the repetitive throwing of a ball or javelin. These "overuse" syndromes are frequently observed in the young female athlete, and include stress fractures, chondromalacia of the patella, certain tendinitis and bursitis conditions, inflammations of fascia such as plantar fascitis, and the ubiquitous "shin splints." The occurrence of a given overuse syndrome in a given athlete at a specific time is usually the result of the interaction of several factors: an error in training, such as too much too fast; an anatomic malalignment of the bones or joints, including the residuals of previous injury; imbalance of the muscle-tendon units of the extremity, either in flexibility or strength; improper equipment, such as ill-fitting running shoes; or running on an improper surface, such as concrete instead of asphalt or dirt [22]. Young female athletes seem to be particularly susceptible to these syndromes. They often lack adequate long-term preparation for vigorous sports training, and because they are often beginning sports training just at the height of the growth spurt, when overgrowth of the bony elements has resulted in a relatively increased tightness of the muscle-tendon units and soft tissue elements of the body, with a secondary loss of flexibility of the joints, young female athletes may be at additional risk for injury.

This combination of inadequate preparation and overgrowth of the muscles and tendons increases the chance of stress injuries occurring. We know that it takes years to condition the bones and soft tissues of the extremities for vigorous athletic activities. Classical ballet, with its rich and long tradition of physical training techniques, requires three or more years of progressive training before a student is allowed advanced technique, including "en pointe."

In the past, the relatively low level of athletic training and physical activity by women in our society rendered them significantly less fit, both cardiovascularily and musculoskeletally, "on the average," than men. While a measurable gain in cardiovascular fitness can take place in a matter of months, with fitness training [9], the musculoskeletal system and, in particular, the bones of the extremities take much longer to remodel and strengthen themselves in response to increased physical demands [22, 26]. We are now seeing two overuse injuries in particular that appear to occur with greater frequency in the young female athlete. These are stress fractures of the lower extremities and patellar problems. Both are also seen in boys, but appear to be occurring more frequently in athletically active girls.

Stress fractures of bone are somewhat analogous to fatigue fractures in metal, with the additional consideration that, in a stress fracture, the body's normal ability to heal microfractures in the bone has been defeated because of the frequency or intensity of the repetitive trauma.

The normal response of bone to increased mechanical stress is to alter its tertiary structure by increasing the number of trabeculae in cancellous bone or the number and alignment of the osteotal systems of cortical bone. If this process occurs gradually and progresssively, significant increase in bony strength can occur. In addition, bone exposed to recurrent microtrauma stress can also increase in overall size, as in the throwing arm of baseball pitchers. We have seen stress fractures in athletes who are at all levels of skill, and the common denominator is usually a significant change in the intensity or frequency of training before the onset of symptoms.

Once again, dramatic comparative data is available from the statistics available at West Point. In the first plebe class with women, of 1976, 10 percent of the young women sustained stress fractures while only 1 percent of the men did. The following year, the summer physical activity program was modified and the incidence of stress fractures was reduced to 3.3 percent in the women. Colonel James L. Anderson, in reviewing this data, commented that "It appears that the higher injury rates for women are largely the result of social cultural bias: these young women have not been acutely culturated to the same demanding physical activity that men are accustomed to. Physiologic stresses they undergo are new to them—to their bones, muscles, and tendons" [2].

The other condition that is seen with high frequency in the young female athlete is chondromalacia patella, or patellofemoral pain syndrome. This, once again, appears to be occurring at a greater rate in the young female athlete than in the young male athlete. Aching pain about the patella with walking or stair climbing, stiffness of the knees with prolonged sitting, or occasional sudden giving way of the knee, are presenting complaints. Although the onset of these complaints may be associated with an error in training or minor injury to the patella, evaluation of an athlete with this complaint will usually show a combination of etiologic factors, the most prominent being imbalance of the musculotendinous units across the knee and the presence of one or more anatomic malalignments of the lower extremity. These anatomic malalignments include femoral anteversion, patella alta, and genu valgum with tibia vara or pes planus.

One of the suggested explanations for the high occurrence of this complaint in young women is the greater width of the female pelvis that, when combined with genu valgum, is said to result in the tendency toward lateral luxation of the patella in the femoral groove [17]. We have found little evidence for this in our patients with this condition, and a survey of growth study films in young male and female patients have shown no significant biomechanical difference in the width of the pelvis or angulation of the tibia and femur at the knee. [20]. We have been much more impressed with muscle-tendon factors such as relative weakness of the quadriceps muscle and tightness of the hamstrings, often in association with the relative growth spurt at the time of initiation of symptoms.

Chondromalacia patella responds well to a conservative program of static straight leg raising (progressive resistance exercises with the knee held in full extension) and musculotendinous flexibility exercises. In addition, orthotic devices placed between the shoe and the foot to alter the foot/ground relationship can often help compensate for anatomic malalignments and at the same time aid in impact absorption. We have found that more than 90 percent of our young female patients with this condition, will respond to conservative techniques [21]. As they increase their level of straight leg weight resistance beyond the 12 to 15 pound range, with ten repetitions, their symptoms slowly but steadily subside.

Once again, it is uncertain whether the apparently increased frequency of this injury in female athletes is the result of a real sexual predisposition or a prior history of low physical activity and subsequent overactivity.

PHYSIOLOGIC DIFFERENCES BETWEEN GIRLS AND BOYS

The traditional concern that girls were at greater risk of injury in sports than boys has been closely associated with concern and observations that girls were less able to sustain the physiologic stress of sports or attain levels of cardiovascular or musculoskeletal fitness similar to boys involved in athletic training.

Until quite recently, it was assumed that girls did not have the stamina for sustained endurance sports such as distance running, swimming, or biking. Certain early studies suggested that aerobic fitness of females was much lower than males [5, 11]. These studies were often comparing individuals at much different levels of training, levels where different demands had been placed on the individuals tested. They did not provide an adequate reflection of the female athletic potential for fitness.

A historic parallel of this concern was the absence of distance running events for girl athletic competitors, including Olympic competition. In the 1928 Olympics, an 800 meter competition was added with only three weeks' notice. Previous maximal distance for women had been 300 meters. A number of the inadequately prepared competitors collapsed without finishing the race, and the subsequent controversy set back women's running competition for a several decades. In the 1984 Olympics, however, women will run the marathon.

Recent studies of cardiovascular fitness and training for women, however, have confirmed that the physiologic response of athletically trained women to endurance stress is very similar to that of their male counterparts and far exceeds that of the untrained, unfit male in our society [11, 25, 33]. Perhaps the coup de grace to this prejudice against women competing in endurance contests is the routine participation of women in the Triathalon—a grueling ordeal consisting of a 2½-

mile swim, followed by a 110-mile bicycle race, and capped by a regulation marathon. There are no breaks between these events.

Other recent longitudinal studies have shown that children, both boys and girls, respond to endurance training in much the same manner as adults [6]. Once again, there appears to be little difference between girls and boys in ability to attain high levels of aerobic fitness in response to endurance training, laying to rest more traditional concerns about the safety of endurance stress for children, and, in particular, girls [4].

MUSCULAR STRENGTH

Another traditional question, and one less easily dismissed, is the differing ability of girls and boys to develop muscular strength. This question has frequently been raised about male and female participation in contact sports, where it has been tacitly assumed that the physically weaker female will be at greater risk of injury than her male opponent or teammate.

It has been well demonstrated that muscle bulk is associated with increased levels of androgens [3, 11]. Weight lifters and body builders have frequently used the muscle-bulking properties of supplemental androgen. There is not, however, a direct correlation between muscle bulk and muscle strength.

Numerous studies have documented the increase in both muscle size and strength in males at puberty, and both have been ascribed to the rising levels of androgens at this stage of development. Conversely, studies of women have shown little if any significant increase in strength at puberty [23]. However, the difference in upper body strength between males and females is much more pronounced than the difference in average lower body strength [11, 19, 23]. This observation has been frequently noted, and relative weakness in upper body strength was one of the most striking observations made of the female plebes at West Point in 1976 [2].

Despite a relatively lower average of muscle strength, particularly in the upper extremities, the female, when exposed to systematic weight training, shows a pattern of strength increase very similar to that of the male [19, 32]. We feel that weight training, properly done, not only improves the athletic performance of the female athlete, but also helps to decrease injury rates in their sports. Unfortunately, many female athletes and dancers have stayed away from weight training because of concern over developing "big" muscles.

Recent studies of this phenomenon have been reassuring. Strength gains from weight training is not accompanied by muscle bulking in most females [11, 32]. It remains to be seen whether the upper limits of attainable weight lifting and strength for the female will match those of the male. However, we must at this time recommend systematic weight training as a safe and protective technique for the young female athlete just as it is for the young male. The strengthened bones, ligaments, and muscle-tendon units have an increased resistance to injury. Systematic weight training for the female athlete is therefore strongly recommended as a supplement to overall athletic training.

As has been noted in other observed differences between male and female athletes, this observed difference in male and female strength may have a social rather than a physical basis. Studies of prepubescent children show no significant difference in motor behavior including strength, reflexes, and endurance between girls and boys [27]. The changes in average strength between boys and girls that occur after puberty have, in the past, been ascribed to the disparate levels of androgens in the postpubescent adults. This does not adequately explain the great differences in upper body strength and the relatively smaller differences in lower body strength between males and females, including male and female athletes [2, 11, 23, 32].

In the past, our society has dictated a significantly different pathway for male and female role development after puberty. In general, the male, and particularly the athletic male, performed much more upper extremity work and muscle training than the female. Boys and girls who were actively climbing trees or playground equipment together at age 9 thereafter often followed different paths. At 13, it was felt quite appropriate for the male to lift weights and the female to watch him.

Conversely, there has been relatively less difference in lower extremity exercise between males and females after puberty. The young women, while learning to "behave like a lady," may have abandoned climbing trees or throwing, but not standing, walking, or running. Thus, a relatively small differential is noted between male and female average lower extremity strength after puberty.

When properly trained male and female athletes of similar size and weight, and even more importantly, of similar lean body mass, were compared, there was an increase in both upper and lower body strength in response to a progressive weight training program that was quite similar [32]. The average levels of muscular strength attained in the male was higher than that of the female and this may indeed be on a sexual or hormonal basis, but much more work is needed in this field before this can be determined with certainty.

One of the bases for the traditional belief that women are weaker than men, and therefore more prone to injury, is the observed differences between performances of male and females in athletics. At the present time, male elite athletes ski faster, swim faster, run faster, and jump higher than female elite athletes. Current athletic records in various sports confirm this. Both individual and team sports have had separate competitions based on sex and many coaches and athletes seem determined to maintain this situation, supporting this stand by citing the "unfairness" of equal competition, or the increased risk of injury in this situation. Ironically, no clear relationship between strength, performance, and injury risk has been demonstrated. While separate competitions may be more enjoyable and comfortable for some participants they may, in the future, be found to be no more safe, and no more fair, than combined competition. At the Olympic level, there is one sport where women and men compete together— the equestrian events. There is no observed difference in injury rate between males and females in these riding events, and certainly, no claims of unfair advantages held by men.

The final issue to be explored in discussing girls' participation in sports is the traditional concern that girls, in particular, are not psychologically geared to the stresses of athletic competition. While long-term studies of the effect of athletic competition on children in general, and girls in particular, are lacking at this time, those short-term studies which have been done have shown no difference between the short-term response of girls and boys to athletic competition. A recent study of how high-level competition effects the personality and adjustment of female athletes is reassuring. The concern that young female athletes will be "defeminized" by the physical and emotional requirements of competition, and that this defeminization results in problems in social and psychological adaptation, appears unwarranted. Ogilvie and McGuire studied elite girl swimmers competing between 1956 and 1970 who attained national championship level [24]. There were 49 participants in all who were available for follow-up and responded to a questionnaire assessing the current status of their social and familiar relationships. These elite competitors appeared to have sustained a high level of social and familial success and felt that their competition had in no way adversely affected their subsequent functioning as adults in professional or male/female relationships. Based upon this study and other observations, it appears that the young girl athlete can sustain the psychological stress of sports competition in a similar fashion to boy competitors, though, for both, excessive pressure may be harmful.

REFERENCES

1. Albohm, M.   How injuries occur in girls sports. *Phys. Sports Med.* 4:46, 1976.
2. Anderson, J. L.   Women's sports and fitness programs at the U.S. Military Academy. *Phys. Sports Med.* 7:72, 1979.
3. Asmussen, E.   Growth in Muscular Strength and Power. In G. L. Rarick (Ed.), *Physical Activity, Human Growth and Development*. New York: Academic, 1973. P. 60.

4. Astrand, P. O., Engstrom, L., and Eriksson, B. Girl swimmers. *Acta Paediatr. Scand.* 147 [Suppl.]:1,1963.
5. Brouha, L. Physiology of training including age and sex differences. *J. Sports Med. and Phys. Fitness* 2:3, 1962.
6. Brown, C. H., Harrower, J. R., and Deeter, M. F. The effect of cross-country running on pre-adolescent girls. *Med. Sci. Sports* 4:1, 1980.
7. Corbitt, R. W., et al. Female athletes. *J. Phys. Ed. and Rec.* 46:45, 1975.
8. Corbitt, R. W., et al. Female athletes. *J.A.M.A.* 228:1266, 1974.
9. Cunningham, D. A., and Hill, J. S. Effects of training on cardiovascular response to exercise in women. *J. Appl. Physiol.* 39:891, 1975.
10. Dale, E., et al. Physical fitness profiles and reproductive physiology of the female distance runner. *Phys. Sports Med.* 7:83, 1979.
11. Drinkwater, B. L. Physiologic response of women to exercise. In *Exercise and Sports Review.* New York: Academic Press, 1973. Vol. 1, p. 126.
12. Erdelyi, G. J. Gynecological survey of female athletes. *J. Sport Med. Phys. Fitness* 2:174, 1972.
13. Frisch, P. E. Fatness and the onset and maintenance of menstrual cycle. *Res. Reprod.* 6:1, 1977.
14. Garrick, J. G., and Regua, R. K. Girl's sports injuries in high school athletics. *J.A.M.A.* 239:2245, 1978.
15. Gehlsen, G., and Albohm, M. Evaluation of sports bras. *Phys. Sports Med.* 8:890, 1980.
16. Gillette, J. When and where women are injured in sports. *Phys. Sports Med.* 3:61, 1975.
17. Haycock, C. E. and Gillette, J. V. Susceptibility of women athletes to injury. *J.A.M.A.* 236:163, 1976.
18. Ingeman, O. Menstruation in Finnish Top Class Sportswomen. In M. J. Karvonen (Ed.), *Sports Medicine.* Helsinki: Finnish Assoc. of Sports Medicine, 1953. P. 96.
19. Mayhew, J. L., and Gross, P. M. Body composition changes in young women with high resistance weight training. *Res. Q. Am. Assoc. Health Phys. Educ.* 45:109, 1974.
20. Micheli, L. J. Personal communication.
21. Micheli, L. J. The Female Runner. In D'Ambrosia and R. and D. Drez (Eds.), *Prevention and Treatment of Running Injuries.* Thorofore, N.J.: Charles B. Slack, 1981.
22. Micheli, L. J., et al. Etiologic assessment of overuse stress fractures in athletes. *Nova Scotia Med. Bull.* 59:43, 1980.
23. Montoye, H. J., and Lamphier, D. E. Grip and arm strength in males and females, age 10 to 69. *Res. Q. Am. Assoc. Health Phys. Educ.* 48:109, 1977.
24. Ogilvie, B. C., and McGuire, L. G. How competition affects elite women swimmers. *Phys. Sports Med.* 8:113, 1980.
25. Plowman, S. Physiological characteristics of female athletes. *Res. Q. Am. Assoc. Health Phys. Educ.* 45:349, 1974.
26. Pollack, M. L., et al. Effects of frequency and duration of training on attrition and incidence of injury. *Med. Sci. Sports* 9:31, 1977.
27. Rarick, G. L., and Dobbins, D. A. Basic components in the motor performance of children six to nine years of age. *Med. Sci. Sports* 7:105, 1975.
28. Sullivan, J. A., et al. Evaluation of injuries in youth soccer. *Am. J. Sports Med.* 8:325, 1980.

29. Ullyot, J. *Women's Running.* Mountain View, Calif.: World Pub. 1977.
30. Vigersky, R. A. et al. Hypothalamus dysfunction in secondary amenorrhea associated with simple weight loss. *N. Engl. J. Med.* 297:1141, 1977.
31. Whitesides, P. A. Men's and women's injuries in comparable sports. *Phys. Sports Med.* 8:130, 1980.
32. Wilmore, J. H. Alterations in strength, body composition, and anthropometric measurements consequent to a 10-week training program. *Med. Sci. Sports* 6:133, 1974.
33. Wilmore, J. H., and Brown, H. C. Physiological profiles of women distance runners. *Med. Sci. Sports* 6:178, 1974.

11. Sports and the Handicapped Child
Robert C. Cantu

The physical disabilties referred to in this chapter include the hereditary and drug-induced birth defects, cerebral palsy, as well as the acquired loss of sight, hearing, or one or more limbs anatomically by amputation or functionally by neurological impairment. While sports mean different things to different people, for most children it provides a pleasurable and purposeful means of using leisure time. For the disabled child, sports may assume a far more significant role as a primary activity and allow them to maximize their participation in the world with their nondisabled peers.

Sports, in addition to providing important social contact, may provide the opportunity to improve muscular function in a particular disability, thus enhancing whatever physiotherapy may have been started. Recreational activities may even accomplish specific functional treatment objectives not attainable with other therapeutic media. Physical motions not possible through routine occupational therapy crafts have been witnessed during games. Of uppermost importance is the keen interest and spirit that sports and games generate, increasing motivation, physical tolerance, and self-confidence when emphasis is taken off the disability and placed on the activity. Indeed, for some handicapped children sports may become the primary motivation for life.

HISTORICAL PERSPECTIVES
Systematic efforts to aid the handicapped date back only about 200 years. During the early years essentially all the pioneers were European. French leaders included Jean Itard, Eduard Sequin, and Alfred Benet. Sign language for the deaf was developed by Abbe Sicard and writing for the blind by Louis Braille. Johann Pestalozzi was a leader in Switzerland, Maria Montessori in Rome, and Alfred Adler and Agust Aickhorn in Austria. One of the early leaders whose philosophical and educational writings provided spiritual impetus was the Swiss-French philosopher Jean Jacques Rousseau.

In the last half century, the United States has become the acknowledged leader in research, services, and programs for children with physical, mental, and emotional disabilities. The economic resources and freedom of investigation in the United States has afforded a climate for unsurpassed growth of theory, research, experimentation, and demonstration projects. Since World War II there has been a marked improvement in public attitudes toward the disabled. This has resulted in new legislation, funding, institutions, and many novel approaches toward treatment of the handicapped child.

PHYSIOLOGY OF EXERCISE FOR THE DISABLED

It has been shown that the physically handicapped through exercise can achieve the same physical and emotional benefits as those of us not so disabled. When fitness test results of a group of wheelchair athletes were compared with those of nonwheelchair athletes, the same increased aerobic capacity and overall training effect was seen for arm work as has been shown for leg work, such as in runners. The wheelchair athletes had significantly higher oxygen uptakes and lower resting and exertional heart rates. Other studies have shown the increased blood flow realized in regularly exercised arms as compared to those not so physically trained. It is clear that, through equivalent aerobic activity using other portions of the body, the handicapped child can realize the same emotional and physical benefits from exercise, within the limits of his or her handicap, as the normal child.

Sports, and in general, participation in the outdoors, may also provide a sense of freedom otherwise unknown to the handicapped child. Imagine the different perspective an otherwise wheelchair-bound paraplegic child has from the saddle of a horse, seat of a kayak shooting the rapids, or from a sailplane soaring high above the earth. Moreover, speaking specifically of sports, aside from the physical benefits of exercise, the emotional "highs" are even greater for the physically handicapped child. The aesthetic enjoyment, opportunity for personal expression, enriching life experience, and therapeutic benefits attained through sports acquires a heightened level for the disabled child.

SELECTION OF A RECREATIONAL PURSUIT

All children have varied personalities, temperaments, and physical characteristics that result in different recreational preferences; the presence of physical disabilty does not change these inherent traits. Whereas most handicapped children can participate in almost all recreational pursuits with special equipment, thought to some special considerations should be given. First, it is important that the particular sport embarked upon provide an opportunity for enjoyment and success while not being especially hazardous because of the specific disability.

It is important to bear in mind the differing needs, experience, and implications of the particular medical affliction rendering the individual handicapped. Certainly the requirements and approach for the congenital paraplegic from a myelomeningocele, the child paraplegic from a car accident, and the paraplegic child with terminal cancer or progressive neurological disease are vastly different. Children recovering from an injury or illness should be guided toward those activities requiring progressively increased physical strength and endurance, while those afflicted with relentlessly progressive illness should be involved with activities they can pursue regardless of diminishing physical activity.

The choice of a sport must reflect the taste of the child, to some extent the type and degree of handicap, and especially his determination and motivation. A flexible approach is required for each child, especially when multiple handicaps, coordination problems and strength deficits complicate the picture. The variation in duration of the handicaps and natural course of the affliction must also be considered.

Money can enter into the picture, as many disabled children have limited financial resources and some sports are quite expensive. The disabled child should be encouraged to adopt the attitude that cost will not prevent their participation in a sport. Given adequate determination and motivation, financial barriers can be overcome as there are numerous monetary resources for special equipment, courses, and other needs for the handicapped.

Specially constructed equipment makes possible virtually all sports for the handicapped child. The key to skiing for the amputee, for instance, is the outrigger. This is a ski tip attached by a hinged mount to an adjustable metal crutch. Amputee skiers use two such outriggers in a manner similar to a crutch, except that when skiing they lean forward on the outriggers for balance. Some outriggers are fitted with a spring-loaded spike that plunges several inches into the snow from the center of the ski. This acts much like a conventional ski pole to afford assistance on the level or uphill. With practice, conditioning, and the outriggers, amazing performances on even the most difficult slalom courses have been achieved.

The unilateral leg amputee who is otherwise in good condition often finds slalom water skiing quite easy to master. Here, only the standard ski is used and no special equipment is required. A trick that aids in reducing the force on the one leg at the start is to lean forward over the ski before the boat accelerates. Once the boat accelerates, the amputee in this position body-planes to the upright position, then stands on the one leg. The increased surface area of the chest aids in having the ski on top of the water more quickly. Water skiing is also enjoyed by the blind as well as the arm amputee.

One might wonder how the lower extremity amputee can sky dive and withstand the impact on landing. This does require planning. The solution is taken from our own as well as Russia's space program. Just as our space craft descends by parachute into the ocean, the amputee sky diver can find a soft landing in a lake, reservoir, or other similar body of water. As the Russians utilize the desert, so, too, a sandpit can serve as an alternative landing site.

Paraplegics and bilateral lower extremity amputees have taken up a variety of activities, many of which this author would be hesitant to try. I can assure you, I have no desire to duplicate the mountain climbing, the rappeling down sheer mountain cliffs, or the parakiting behind a speeding car, exploits enjoyed by uni- and bilateral leg amputees. These are sports that many "normal" people cannot perform, so we must understand that the word *cripple* is of extremely limited (and quite probably, no) value.

Scuba diving presents no problem when a special shortened wet suit is worn with flippers firmly attached to the suit legs just below the stumps. Sailing, sledding, canoeing, angling, rock climbing, caving, hang-gliding, and even wheelchair parakiting behind a moving car have been reported. Horseback riding can be enjoyed by the bilateral amputee with or without prostheses. A safety belt similar to those used in automobiles can be employed to hold the rider in the saddle. Riding is also a favorite activity of and therapy for many suffering from mental illness; cerebral palsy; congenital, hereditary, neurological, and traumatic conditions; and the blind, deaf, and limbless. While some may not progress beyond walking on a horse, others will acquire new skills and freedom and be able to join leisure activities on a par with able-bodied riders. Regardless of skill, all experience a feeling of freedom and independence. While riding, they can essentially forget their physical disability and, regardless of the terrain, go where they want. The outdoor feel of sun and wind on the face, the sights, sounds, and smells provide immense enjoyment. Physical benefits besides aerobic exercise include stretching of tight structures, improvement in balance, coordination, body awareness, agility, and relaxation. The element of danger is also present that most disabled children frequently have lacking in their lives and find immensely stimulating.

Today, riding therapy has assumed a major role in the treatment of children with physical, emotional, and intellectual handicaps. Elsebet Bodtker of Norway, a trained physiotherapist, is a recognized pioneer in this field. Recognizing the unique therapeutic values of horseback riding both in developing physical skills and in gaining confidence, she started the world's first riding school for disabled children in 1953. Twenty years later in 1973, the school hosted a world conference on riding therapy. Only very recently has the United States given riding therapy wide acceptance. However, the Cheff Center for the Handicapped located in Augusta, Michigan, is the world's largest riding school. This center has also published an enthusiastically accepted excellent training manual on therapeutic riding for the handicapped.

The disabled rider may participate in riding clubs, especially on the social and organizational side. They can easily assist at horse shows by judging and in many other ways. Finally, there are carefully graded competitions for the disabled. The Scandinavian countries devised these competitions that have been widely copied.

The water sports have their own special attraction that many disabled children find as the best outlet for their abilities. Some of those safely pursued by the handicapped include fly, float, and deep sea fishing, canoeing, kyacking, rowing, sculling, sailing, water skiing, power boating, snorkeling, and, as previously discussed, scuba diving.

It is unfortunate that the potential benefits to be derived by the disabled child from water sports is not more widely recognized. Fishing can be as simple or complicated as the angler wishes it to be. Enjoyed from either a wheelchair or deck chair, it provides a thrilling awareness of the natural environment. A harness or fixed vice-type pole-holder allows for one-handed fishing. Special lightweight rods, spinning reels, and other special devices for the handicapped fisherman are available through catalogues and customer service personnel from several companies including the Orvis Company, L. L. Bean, and Abercrombie and Fitch. Sailing and canoeing contain more of a risk element that most youngsters find very stimulating.

It is the awareness of a new sense of freedom that is perhaps the greatest reward experienced by the disabled children who participate in water sports. For those with restricted movement, such involvement is like living in another dimension where the difficulties in walking can be forgotten.

Today in the late twentieth century, we live in an era of supersophisticated technology, and for the disabled, this can be especially beneficial. Target shooting for quadraplegics illustrates one of the most technical, competitive recreational pursuits for the handicapped. Two physicians from the Sheba Medical Center, Tel-Hashomer, Israel devised a new flexible spring-coil, multi-directional mounting device enabling competitive target shooting for individuals with severe bilateral upper and lower extremity physical handicaps, and they even developed rules based on severity of quadraplegia. This devise thus affords the quadraplegic child the opportunity and satisfaction in participating in yet another sport.

Of all the disabled, amputees have perhaps the widest range of sports activities. Indeed, a single, especially partial upper limb, amputee is little disabled for running, race-walking, speed-skating, throwing the javelin or shot-put, ping-pong, and a number of other pursuits (see Table 11-3). As regards lower limb amputees, below-knee amputees are significantly more independent than above-knee and bilateral amputees. There is essentially no difference between above-knee and bilateral amputees. Lower limb amputees listed fishing and swimming among the most popular recreational activities, while running and walking long distances head the list of most arduous.

For the paraplegic child, the wheelchair becomes their "wheels." Organized competitions in archery, basketball, badminton, bowling, croquet, darts, fencing, discus, golf, horseshoes, ping-pong, pool, riflery, and road races including marathons, have all been arranged. Other leisure pursuits from square dancing to gardening are enjoyed from the wheelchair seat. It is recommended that wheelchairs being used for outdoor sports have removable arms, swinging or removable footrests, antitrip levers, outer hand rims, and, when desired, pneumatic tires.

For those who become deeply interested in competition, the International Sports for the Disabled (see Athletic Organizations for the Disabled at the end of this chapter) sponsors meets regularly held on a regional, national, and international level. The National Wheelchair Games (U.S.) and International Paralympics are held annually with events including shot-put, wheelchair track dashes and relays, weight-lifting, archery, table tennis, swimming and basketball.

The International Sports for the Disabled aims to not only unite in international cooperation national groups to encourage further development of sports programs, but to provide a forum for the exchange of opinions, experiences, and resources related to sports for the disabled. It also prepares and disseminates international standards so that individuals are divided into disability classifications to permit fair competition between participants with similar degrees of handicaps. Groups are classified as:

Class I   Complete spinal paraplegia at T_9 or above, or comparable disability where there is a total loss of muscular function originating at T_{11} or above.

Class I-A   Incomplete quadriplegia. Incomplete paralysis of upper extremities, with involvement of trunk and paralysis of the lower extremities.

Class II   Complete spinal paraplegia at T_{10} or below, or comparable disability where there is a significant loss of muscular function of hips and thighs.

Class III   All other disabilities.

HOW TO ARRANGE AN EXERCISE PROGRAM

The basic requirements of an exercise program for the disabled child is the same as that for the nondisabled. Each exercise program should have three parts: a warm-up, an endurance phase, and a cooling-off period.

The *warm-up* phase should be at least five minutes and include rhythmic slow stretching movements of the trunk and limb muscles. This increases blood flow and stretches the postural muscles preparing the body for sustained activity. To ignore the warm-up is to risk muscle-pulls or more severe injuries.

The *cooling-off* phase is too often omitted in exercise. While the endurance phase significantly raises body temperature, increases the heart rate and blood pressure, and builds up lactic acid and other waste products in your muscles, the cooling-off phase allows the bodily functions to gradually return to normal. This helps to eliminate waste products from the muscles, minimizing the chance of stiffness and soreness the next day. The cooling-off phase should last at least five minutes and can be longer if desired. It should include gross body movements that emphasize range of motion of the joints. Calisthenics are ideal for this final step in the day's exercise program.

The *endurance* phase should last at least 30 minutes. During this period, the cardiovascular system is stressed to increase aerobic capacity. To achieve maximal cardiovascular improvement, the child should exercise vigorously enough during the endurance phase to be breathing deeply, but not so vigorously as to fall into greater oxygen debt (gasping for air). As aerobic capacity increases, the time and intensity of the endurance phase may be increased.

For the main endurance phase, I have prepared three tables that list recreational pursuits especially well adapted to the upper limb disabled (Table 11-1), lower limb disabled (Table 11-2), and both upper and lower limb disabled (Table 11-3). Those activities for which 30 minutes of continuous pursuit is sufficient are noted with an asterisk, while those less strenuous requiring an hour or more are not so designated. Activities for the wheelchair-bound are followed by a "W" in parentheses. It must be realized, though, that these tables are neither complete nor exclusive. Given burning motivation and desire,

Table 11-1. Recreational Pursuits Especially
Appropriate for the Upper-Limb Disabled

Backpacking	Platform tennis
Badminton	Riding
*Bicycling	Rodeo
Bowling	*Roller skating
*Cross-country running	*Running
Darts	Snowshoeing
Fencing	*Soccer
*Ice hockey	*Squash
*Ice skating	Tennis
*Jogging	*Track
*Jumping	*Trampoline
Karate	Tumbling
Lawn bowling	Walking
Ping-pong	

Table 11-2. Recreational Pursuits Especially
Appropriate for the Lower-Limb Disabled

Archery (W)	Lawn bowling (W)
*Badminton (W)	Motocross
Baseball (W)	Motorcycling
*Basketball (W)	Ping-Pong (W)
Boating (W)	Pool (W)
Body building (W)	*Rowing (W)
Bowling (W)	Sailplanes
*Canoeing	Show jumping
Folk-dancing (W)	Softball (W)
Football (touch or flag) (W)	*Sculling
Gliding	Tobogannning
Golf (W)	*Volleyball (W)
*Handball (W)	Weight lifting (W)
*Kayaking	

Table 11-3. Recreational Pursuits Enjoyed
by Upper- and Lower-Limb Disabled

Alpine skiing	Ice fishing
*Body surfing	Isometrics
Bowling	Ping-pong
Calisthenics	Rock climbing
Camping	Sailing
*Cross-country skiing	Scuba diving
Dancing	Skin diving
Diving (platform)	Skydiving
Fishing	Snorkeling
Gardening	Sports car rallying
Gymnastics	*Swimming
Hiking	Target shooting
Horseback riding	*Water-skiing
Hunting	

with ingenuity and equipment, there is virtually no sport, from scuba diving to sky diving, that today the disabled child cannot master and enjoy. Following are some of the many athletic organizations for the disabled child, as well as a selected bibliography.

ATHLETIC ORGANIZATIONS FOR THE DISABLED

THE BLIND

Blind Outdoor Leisure Development (Founded: 1969)
533 E. Main Street
Aspen, Colorado 81611
Phone: (303) 925-8922
Richard C. Fenton, Executive Director
Operates on the "can-do" theory for blind people. Aids in the establishment of local clubs in order to enable the blind to experience the

out-of-doors by skiing, skating, camping, and biking. Designs and conducts training courses for activity leaders; has designed distinctive jackets and bibs to identify participants as blind; provides insurance program for participants. Local clubs solicit reduced costs for or free use of sports equipment and facilities.

British Association for Sporting and Recreational Activities For The Blind
1 Malvern Close
Prestwich
Manchester, England

National Association of Visually Handicapped Bowlers
23 Bolnant Avenue
Leicester, England

THE DEAF

American Athletic Association For the Deaf (Founded: 1945)
3916 Lantern Drive
Silver Springs, Maryland 20902
Phone: (301) 942-4042
Richard Caswell, Secretary-Treasurer
To foster athletic competition among the deaf and regulate uniform rules governing such competition; to provide adequate competition for those members who are primarily interested in interclub athletics; to provide a social outlet for deaf members and their friends. Sanctions and promotes state, regional, and national basketball tournaments, softball tournaments, participation in activities of the Committee International des Sports Silencieux and in World Games for the Deaf. Maintains AAAD Hall of Fame and gives annual Athlete of the Year Award. *Publications:* Bulletin, quarterly. *Convention/Meeting:* Semi-annual—always April and September. 1979 Houston, Texas, and Cleveland, Ohio; 1980 San Diego, California, and Indianapolis, Indiana; 1981 Buffalo, New York, and Hartford, Connecticut; 1982 Miami, Florida, and Vancouver, British Columbia, Canada.

International Committee of the Silent Sports (Founded: 1924)
Gallaudet College
Washington, D.C. 20002
Phone: (202) 447-0841
Jerald M. Jordan, Executive Secretary
Membership composed of athletic organizations for the deaf in each of 43 countries. Provides an international sports competition for the deaf, patterned after the Olympic Games. Seeks to promote and develop physical education in general, and the practice of sports in particular, among the deaf; encourages friendly relations between countries with programs in silent sports and formation of silent sports

programs in countries not yet participating. Holds Summer World Games and Winter Games alternately at two-year intervals. All competitors must have severe hearing loss. Awards gold, silver, and bronze metals to first, second, and third place winners of each event. Medals recognizing valuable personal contribution to the Committee are also awarded. The Committee is recognized by the International Olympic Committee. *Publications:* (1) Bulletin, quarterly; (2) Handbook, irregular. *Convention/Meeting:* Biennial congress—held concurrently with Games.

International Games For The Deaf (Founded: 1924)
Langaavel 41
DK-2650 Hvidovre, Denmark
Knud Sondergaard, Secretary-General
National associations for deaf sports united to: develop and control the physical education in general and the practice of sports in particular among the deaf of the world; encourage relations between the countries practicing sports for the deaf; initiate and then give guidance to the practice of sports in countries where this is unknown; supervise the regular celebration of the World Games for the Deaf. Conduct quadrennial World Games for the Deaf. *Publications:* (1) Bulletin (includes directory), quarterly; (2) Yearbook, every eight years. *Affiliated with:* International Olympic Committee. *Convention/Meeting:* Biennial— 1979—Meribel, France; 1981 Tehran, Iran.

United States Deaf Skiers Association (Founded: 1968)
159 Davis Avenue
Hackensack, New Jersey 07601
Dan Fields, President
Promotes skiing, both recreational and competitive, among the deaf and hearing-impaired in the United States. Provides deaf skiers benefits, activities and opportunities that will further increase their enjoyment of the sport. Encourages ski-racing among the deaf and sponsors national and regional races for deaf skiers. Assists in any way possible the selection, organization and training of the United States Deaf Ski Teams for international competition, such as hockey for the World Winter Games for the Deaf. Presents awards. *Committees:* Ice Figure Skating; Speed Skating. *Publications:* Newsletter, 4/year. *Affiliated with:* United States Ski Association. *Convention/Meeting:* Biennial—1980 February, Steamboat Springs, Colorado; 1982 Big Sky, Montana.

British Deaf Sports Council
25 Hallfield Road
Bradford
West Yorkshire BD1 3RD England

THE PARALYZED AND AMPUTEES

International Sports Organization For The Disabled (ISOD) (Founded: 1963)
Stoke Mandeville Sports Stadium
Harvey Road
Aylesbury, Buckinghamshire, England
Joan Scruton, Secretary-General
National organization in 27 countries concerned with development of sports for the disabled. Sponsors international seminars for training and education; coordinates international activities of members. *Convention/Meeting:* Biennial Olympiad for the Physically Disabled in conjunction with the International Stoke Mandeville Games Federation.

International Stoke Mandeville Games Federation
Stoke Mandeville Sports Stadium
Harvey Road
Aylesbury, Buckinghamshire, England
Joan Scruton, Secretary-General
National organizations concerned with development of sports for paralyzed individuals. Organizes annual International Stoke Mandeville Games (Olympics of the Paralyzed), which are held for three consecutive years at the Stoke Mandeville Sports Stadium and every fourth year in the country of the Olympic Games. *Publications:* The Cord, three times a year.

National Foundation For Happy Horsemanship For The Handicapped (Founded: 1967)
Box 462
Malvern, Pennsylvania 19355
Phone: (215) 644-7414
Maudie Hunter-Warfel, National Advisor
Individuals who assist handicapped persons in their involvement with horses as a form of therapy and rehabilitation. Purpose is to encourage and unify the teaching of driving horses to the disabled through the training of personnel for this, and the arranging of exchanges among those who have experience in the field. Experience has shown that involvement with horses can do much for the handicapped person by reducing their concentration on self and disillusionment with life. Provides horses and donates facilities for their care. *Publications:* Newsletter, annual. *Convention/Meeting:* Biennial—1979 September, England.

National Handicapped Sports and Recreation Association (Founded: 1972)
4105 E. Florida Ave., Third Fl.
Denver, Colorado 80222
Phone: (303) 232-4575

Fred T. Nichol, President
Amputees and other handicapped persons who are interested in participating in all kinds of sports. To provide veterans and other inconvenienced (handicapped) persons an opportunity to experience sports and participatory recreation activities. Sponsors ski clinics and publishes an amputee ski technique manual. *Publications:* Bulletin, semiannual; also publishes Amputee Ski Technique Manual and Blind Ski Teaching Manual. *Formerly:* (1972) National Amputee Skiers Association; (1977) National Inconvenienced Sportsmen's Assoc. *Convention/ Meeting:* Annual.

National Wheelchair Athletic Association (Founded: 1958)
2107 Templeton Gap Road, Suite C
Colorado Springs, Colorado 80907
Phone: (303) 632-0698
D. Dale Wiley, Chairman
Men and woman athletes with significant permanent neuromuscular-skeletal disability (spinal cord disorder, poliomyelitis, amputation) who compete in various amateur sports events in wheelchairs. The Association is administered by, and under the jurisdiction of, the National Wheelchair Athletic Committee. Members compete in regional events and in the annual National Wheelchair Games, which include competitions in track and field (including pentathalon), swimming, archery, table tennis, slalom and weightlifting. Qualifying rounds are held in each region to select competitors for the national competition. Selection is made at the completion of the nationals to represent the U.S. team in international competition. Travel expenses for the U.S. competitors are subsidized by the U.S. Wheelchair Sports Fund. *Publications:* Newsletter.

National Wheelchair Basketball Association (Founded: 1958)
110 Seaton Bldg.
University of Kentucky
Lexington, Kentucky 40506
Phone: (606) 257-1623
Stan Labanowich, Ph.D., Commissioner
Wheelchair basketball teams made up of individuals with severe permanent physical disabilities of the lower extremities. Seeks to provide opportunities on a national basis for the physically disabled to participate in the sport of wheelchair basketball, with its adjunct psychological, social, and emotional benefits, and to maintain a high level of competition through continuing refinement and standardization of playing rules and officiating. Sponsors competitions, maintains Hall of Fame, compiles statistics, participates in charitable activities. Awards trophy annually to winner of National Wheelchair Basketball Tour-

nament. *Publications:* (1) Weekly Standings and Statistics (November–April); (2) Newsletter, biweekly (November–April); (3) Casebook, annual; (4) Directory, annual; (5) National Wheelchair Basketball Tournament Program, annual; (6) Rule Book, annual. *Convention/Meeting:* Annual sectional and regional tournaments leading up to the national tournament.

North American Riding For The Handicapped Association (Founded: 1968)
c/o Leonard Warner
P.O. Box 100
Ashburn, Virginia 22011
Phone: (703) 777-3540
Leonard Warner, Secretary-Treasurer
Individuals and centers for the handicapped. Seeks to promote therapeutic riding for the handicapped with good safety and proper care; to provide appropriate training and certification for instructors working with the handicapped. Makes periodic inspections of riding centers in operation. Provides consultants as lecturers and demonstrators. *Publications:* Newsletter, annual.

Special Olympics (Founded: 1968)
1701 K St., N.W., Suite 203
Washington, D.C. 20006
Phone: (202) 331-1346
Eunice Kennedy Shriver, President
Created and sponsored by the Joseph P. Kennedy, Jr. Foundation to promote physical education and athletics for the retarded. Local, area, and chapter games are conducted in 50 states, District of Columbia, Puerto Rico, and 24 foreign countries. International Special Olympics are staged quadrennially (next 1983). Participants range in age from 8 years to adult and compete in track and field, swimming, gymnastics, bowling, ice skating, basketball, and other sports. Information materials are available on organization of programs and participation of athletes. Presents annual awards for service to program through sports. Maintains speakers bureau; compiles statistics; sponsors research program. *Councils:* National Advisory. *Publications:* (1) Newsletter (restricted circulation), quarterly; (2) List of Chapter and National Directors, annual; also publishes brochure, guide, instructional manual and list of state programs. *Convention/Meeting:* Annual conference of chapter and national directors.

ADDITIONAL READING

Adapted Sports in Veterans Administration. Special Service Information Bulletin 1B 6-252. Recreation Service, V.A., Washington, D.C.
Barnett, M. W. Blind girl in the troop. *Girl Scout Leader.* April, 1966. P. 20.

Barnett, M. W.   *Handicapped Girls and Girl Scouting. A Guide for Leaders.* New York: Girl Scouts of the United States of America, 1968.

Bauman, M. D., and Strausse, S.   A comparison of blind children from day and residential schools in a camp setting. *Int. J. Educ. Blind* 11:74, 1962.

Becker, E. F.   *Female Sexuality Following Spinal Cord Injury.* Accent Spinal Pub. Chever Pub. Inc., P.O. Box 700, Bloomington, Ill.: 61701.

Buell, C. E.   Developments in physical education for blind children. *New Outlook Blind* 58:202, 1964.

Buell, C. E.   *Physical Education for Blind Children.* Springfield, Ill.: Thomas, 1966.

Dendy, E.   Recreation for disabled people—what do we mean. *Physiotherapy* 64:290, 1978.

Emes, C.   Physical work capacity of wheelchair athletes. *Res. Q. Am. Assoc. Health Phys. Educ.* 48:209, 1977.

Frampten, M. E., and Mitchell, P. C.   *Camping for Blind Youth.* New York: American Institute for the Education of the Blind, 1949.

Ginglend, D., and Gould, K.   *Day Camping for the Mentally Retarded.* New York: National Assoc. for Retarded Children, 1962.

Guide to Fishing Facilities for Disabled Anglers. National Anglers Council, 5 Cowgate, Peterborough, PEI ILR, Canada, 1978.

Holidays for the Physically Handicapped. Royal Assoc. for Disability and Rehabiltation Annual 1978 edition.

Howe, G. T.   Canoe course for the blind. *Recreation* 55:131, 1962.

Howett, H. H. (Ed.)   *Camping for Crippled Children.* Chicago: National Society for Crippled Children and Adults, 1945.

Juul, K. D.   European approaches and innovations in serving the handicapped. *Except. Child* 44:322, 1978.

Kapurch, J. A.   Camping though handicapped. *Am. J. Nurs.* 66:1794, 1966.

Kegel, B., Carpenter, M. D., and Burgess, E. M.   Functional capabilities of lower extremity amputees. *Arch. Phys. Med. Rehab.* 59:109, 1978.

Kirchman, M. M.   Rifle holder. *Am. J. Occup. Ther.* 19:28, 1965.

Meyers, T.   *Camping for Emotionally Disturbed Boys.* Bloomington: Indiana University Department of Recreation; School of Health, Physical Education and Recreation, 1961.

Mooney, H. V.   Fabricating of fin prostheses for bilateral amputee. *Ortho. Prosth. Appl. J.* September, 20: 221, 1966.

Paraplegia Life. Published by National Spinal Cord Injury Foundation, 369 Elliot St., Newton Upper Falls, Mass. 02164.

Rathbone, J. L., and Lucus, C.   *Recreation in Total Rehabilitation.* Springfield, Ill.: Thomas, 1959.

Recreation for disabled people. *Physiotherapy* 64:299, 1978.

Schoenbohm, W. F.   *Planning and Operating Facilities for Crippled Children.* Springfield, Ill.: Thomas, 1962.

Sports and Spokes. 4330 East-West Highway, Suite 300, Washington, D.C. 20014.

Stewart, F.   *Recreation for the Retarded, A Handbook for Leaders.* Nat. Soc. of Mentally Handicapped Children, Pembridge Hall, Pembridge Square, London: W2 4EP, 1975.

"State of the Art" on National Recreational Boating for the Physically Handicapped. Human Resource Center, Albertson, Long Island, NY 11507.

Summer camps for deaf children. *Volta Rev.* 64:192, 1962.

Switzer, R. M. and Clark, M.   Camping for severely disabled children. *Interclinic Inform. Bull.*, 1964.

Taggie, J. M., and Manley, M. S. *A Handbook on Sexuality After Spinal Cord Injury.* Family Service Dept., Craig Hospital, 3425 S. Clarkson St., Englewood, Colo. 80010.

Wakim, K. G., et al. The effects of therapeutic exercise on peripheral circulation of normal and paraplegic individuals. *Arch. Phy. Med. Rehab.* 30:86, 1949.

Walker, G. M. Riding for the disabled. *Physiotherapy* 64:297, 1978.

Water Sports for the Disabled. The Sports Council Advisory Panel. Royal Yachting Association, Victoria Way, Woking, Surrey GU 21 IEQ, England, 1977.

12. Flexibility and Conditioning in the Young Athlete

John S. Leard

Many injuries that occur to athletes could be prevented with proper conditioning programs. A great number of injuries seen at the Division of Sports Medicine at Children's Hospital Medical Center in Boston are caused by some type of overuse or microtrauma. The athlete has usually performed a stressful acvitity that his body was not capable of withstanding. A conditioning program provides a time during which ligaments, musculotendinous units, and bone will adapt to the stress of a new activity.

Conditioning programs will be discussed from three different aspects: muscular strengthening, flexibility, and energy source development [17]. Each of these will be discussed, reviewing general principles and goals. Specific tests for screening and exercise programs will follow.

MUSCULAR STRENGTHENING

In the young athlete, optimum flexibility and strength is essential to decrease injuries and increase performance. Strength is developed by stressing the body over a period of time so adaptations take place in the musculoskeletal system, which will protect itself from this added stress. This is known as the overload principle. It is used both in weight lifting and energy source development where optimum resistance or intensity of activity is gradually increased as the athlete improves his capabilities to perform the task [17].

This adaptation to stress also occurs in the skeletal system and is known as Wolff's Law [26]. The internal conformation and external shape of a bone changes with any constant change in the stress applied, so that it will be best adapted mechanically to resist the stress. When this change in conformation is slower than the amount of constant increased stress on the bone, stress fractures result. Often this type of injury plagues runners who change their running program too quickly. Sometimes a simple change in running surface or shoes will be enough to cause stress fractures. Common areas where these occur are in the tibia, fibula, proximal femur, acetabulum, and metatarsals [20]. Specific weight training will help to avoid these injuries. Increase of muscular strength will help protect the bone and other joint structures. Using the overload principle, optimum muscular, ligamentous, and bone strength is attainable [10].

The suggested method of weight lifting for children is to use the 7–11 system. This system is carried out in four steps:

1. Optimum weight should be found that can be lifted for 3 sets of 7 repetitions in proper form.
2. The number of repetitions are increased until 3 sets of 11 repetitions are attained using the original amount of weight.
3. Now the weight is increased to the maximum weight that can be lifted 3 sets of 7 repetitions.
4. Repeat step 2.

Weight training of a particular muscle group should occur at least every other day, allowing rest and avoiding fatigue of the muscle [16]. Fatigue is a condition of the musculoskeletal system resulting when optimum intensity of training is performed over too long a period of time, or too close in succession. The exhaustion of the muscle energy supplies causes incoordination and a decrease in the intensity of activity. Optimum strength development will not be achieved when this occurs. Optimum effort must take place for strength to develop at its optimum rate [9].

THE LENGTH-TENSION RELATIONSHIP

The length-tension relationship must be considered when referring to optimum muscular effort. The maximum torque that a muscle can develop varies with the position of the joint and the angle of pull of the prime mover of the action. For example, in a bicep curl with weights (this is executed with weight in hand, arm at side, bringing the palm of the hand to the anterior shoulder), the torque developed by the muscle is maximal between 45 and 90 degrees of flexion. Using free weights, the highest amount of weight that may be lifted will be the maximum torque at full extension, when the muscle cannot develop as much torque [21]. This does not mean that lifting with free weight is not beneficial and should not be used to strengthen muscles. This does point out, however, that it may be desirable to perform exercises that vary resistance throughout the range of movement. This should always be done with supervision of someone experienced in weight training. The muscle can contract either isometrically (the muscle contracts but there is no joint motion) or isotonically (the joint moves with muscle contraction). The isotonic contraction can either be concentric (origin toward insertion) or eccentrically (origin away from insertion) [3].

One type of isotonic weight training device is the Universal machine. This involves lifting weights using a pulley system to safely isolate some muscle groups. The machine is convenient and has many stations so a number of athletes can be exercising at the same time. Some of the machines offered by Universal Gym have a dynamic variable resistance that tries to vary resistance to the motion parameters and biomechanical changes of the muscles [25].

There are other types of equipment that attempt to distribute maximum resistance throughout the range of motion. The Nautilus machines and Isokinetic devices are two types of equipment which attempt to do this. The Nautilus works with cam-like gears and pulley systems. The machines are designed to strengthen certain muscle groups and duplicate their length-tension relationship. Another feature of the Nautilus machine is that it gives resistance in all positions throughout a full range of possible movement [24].

Isokinetic devices use a hydraulic system that is set to a certain speed. No matter how hard the athlete pushes, the machine will move at the preset speed. If the athlete pushes as hard and as fast as he or she can, then optimum resistance will be attained throughout the range of motion [23].

WEIGHT TRAINING MYTHS

Over the years, many myths have developed concerning weight training and its effect on athletic performance. Examples range from baseball pitchers not lifting because it will make them tight so they will not throw the ball effectively to long distance runners losing their endurance due to weight training with their legs. The following are six common myths concerning weight training and their rebuttals.

Weight training decreasing endurance has been a favorite myth with some coaches. However, studies reviewed by H. Harrison Clarke have shown that endurance is increased with strength increases by isotonic exercises [5].

Another myth says that flexibility is decreased with weight training. This is not true if weight training is done properly through the entire range of motion and preceded and followed with flexibility exercises. Specific types of stretches will be discussed in the next section.

The third myth states that weight lifting performed with quick, explosive movements is more effective than slow movements. Using weights or weight machines that have no speed control are more beneficial to increasing total muscular strength if they are used at a slow pace without momentum. If the weight is moved quickly, the muscle will be strengthened in the initial range where the explosive contraction occurs. The remaining range will not have as much resistance to the movement than a slower motion because the weight is being propelled and less muscular force is needed to move the weight. The end of the range of motion will have optimum resistance since the weight will be slowed down and held there by the muscle contracting. For overall muscular strength training, a slower movement is more beneficial. The exception to the rule is when weight training is done for an explosive event such as the javelin or shot put. Even with these events, if the youngster is early in his "career," it is better to have basic overall strength before specific weight training is begun.

A fourth myth states that weight training will slow reflexes and reaction time. Discussing this from the point of view of muscle fiber types, "fast twitch" or "slow twitch," we will use the works of Saltin, who showed that muscle fibers are selectively recruited by the activity taking place [27]. The slow twitch fibers are activated at low work rates, and fast twitch fibers are activated in very intensive work loads and at activities requiring high rate of contraction. This negates the myth that weight training will slow reflexes or reaction time since fast twitch fibers are developed in weight training and are used with motions requiring quick movements.

Another myth states that weight training should never be performed during the season of the sport the athlete is playing. Weight training should be performed to maintain the strength that was developed in the off season. Often, the sport will not maintain the strength and flexibility that was developed since it does not consistently stress the body to such a high level. It is suggested that weight training be continued unless performance is decreased from the added exercise. Coaches should allow time in practice sessions for weight training to take place [5].

The last myth to be discussed holds that weight training will increase muscle definition in females to the same extent as males. Muscle bulk or hypertrophy occurs when forceful muscular activity occurs. The diameter of the individual muscle fibers increase and the fibers gain in total number of myofibrils as well as in various nutrient and intermediary substances, such as adenosine triphosphate (ATP), phosphocreatine (PC), and glycogen. This occurs in both males and females. Muscular definition occurs in men due to the male hormone testosterone, which is secreted at puberty. Unless high amounts are present in the female, muscular definition will not occur to the same extent with weight training [9].

THE WEIGHT TRAINING PROGRAM

In all weight training programs, the athlete must constantly be reminded he or she is not weight lifting. Weight lifting is an Olympic event that takes years of weight training to be able to perform. The emphasis in weight training should be the proper form rather than the amount of weight lifted. Competition between lifters to have maximum effort achieved is beneficial as a coaching technique as long as it is not overemphasized. Penalties for improper form when lifting should be used in the weight room, as well as having incentives for the amount lifted.

When developing a weight lifting program, the muscle groups, types of contraction, and speed of movement for the majority of the time during the sport activity have to be evaluated and incorporated into the weight program. Isometric and isotonic strength can be developed either separately or together but should be thought of as two different types of muscular strengths [1]. The strength of the individual and availability of equipment also determines the overall program. One may fully realize what should be done but is unfortunately limited in his or her ability to carry through due to lack of equipment or other circumstances.

Weight training can cause injuries as well as prevent them. Proper technique and simple safety procedures should be told to the athlete and strictly enforced. Free weight, Nautilus, Universal, and Isokinetic devices should be used only after proper instruction and supervision is provided. Details of some suggested free weight training exercises are set forth at the end of this chapter.

FLEXIBILITY

Flexibility exercises should be performed before and after any exercise, whether it is weight training or running. Stretching is thought to prepare the muscle for activity. Stretching will also ensure that strength and flexibility will be developed throughout the entire range of movement. Injuries are more likely to occur if a person is flexible and without strength, or the other extreme, strong and inflexible. In the conditioning program, optimum flexibility and strength should be the goal. The earlier the age flexibility exercises are incorporated into a program, the easier it will be to remain flexible. In growing children, bones often will grow much faster than muscles will stretch. As a result, during the growth spurts near puberty, the body will become relatively inflexible [11, 13, 15]. By performing stretching exercises consistently, flexibility should be maintained and injuries prevented. The types of injuries prevented do not necessarily have to be of the musculotendinous type due to excessive tightness. At the Division of Sports Medicine at Children's Hospital Medical Center in Boston, inflexibility is now being thought of as the primary cause of many overuse injuries. Tightness of the structures in the popliteal area preventing full knee extension are often characteristic of young athletes with chondromalacia. Decreased movement and weakness in the shoulder girdle will sometimes be the predisposing factor causing "little league elbow" or "tennis elbow." Often tightness developed in the hip flexors, hamstrings, and lumbosacral areas during growth as a child results in chronic low back pain caused by improper posture. Continuation of this overuse will sometimes lead to stress fractures of lumbar vertebrae or spondylolysis. Flexibility is not a general property equally apparent in all joints of the individual. Several studies have given evidence that flexibility is specific to the different joints of the body [6, 8, 11, 20]. There are many different joint structures that can cause a decrease in range of motion: ligaments, joint capsule, musculotendinous units, joint surface, etc. The one factor that can most easily be changed to increase motion is muscular tightness.

BASIC STRETCHING MANEUVERS

There are basically three different ways to stretch musculotendinous units: static, modified proprioceptive neuromuscular facilitation (PNF), and ballistic stretch. The static type places the muscle in an elongated position and holds the position. When the muscle relaxes, more stretch is gradually applied. The ballistic stretch elongates the muscle similar to the static method except the athlete bounces, vigorously stretching the muscle to gain more motion.

The method of PNF was developed from Herman Kabat over a period of 5 years, 1946–1951. The PNF Technique was developed further by Knott and Voss in 1956 [14], and uses basic neurophysiological properties of muscle to gain range of movement. They are successive induction, fatigue, and reciprocal induction.

Successive Induction

This is a normal neuromuscular reflex action. Following voluntary contraction of the agonist, the antagonist is facilitated for contraction [12].

Reciprocal Induction

This condition is defined as occurring when the agonist is facilitated and the antagonist is inhibited from contracting [12]. Please note the timing of relaxation and facilitation in these two muscular responses.

Techniques of Relaxation

These techniques utilize maximal contractions of the antagonist (tight muscle) followed by voluntary relaxation, which, whenever possible, is followed by resisted contraction of the agonist [14].

The ballistic stretch should not be performed due to the danger of muscle tearing and the facilitation of the stretch reflex in muscles. By elongating a tight muscle and quickly stretching it, there is the tendency of the muscle to be torn rather than gradually stretched. This quick stretching will also facilitate the spinal reflex causing a readiness of the tight muscle to contract. Quite simply, by quick stretching the tight muscle it becomes tighter rather than more flexible [2].

When performing flexibilities the general guidelines to follow are:

1. Be specific—know what you are trying to stretch and where you should feel the stretch before you begin.
2. The stretch should be performed with a slow gradual movement trying to relax the muscle.

3. There should be no pain while performing the exercise, only the stretching sensation. Be certain the child is aware of this. Pain will lead to overstretching and loss of flexibility.
4. The low back should be protected. Always try to keep the back straight, not arched, when stretching. Obviously, this rule is not followed when specifically stretching the low back.
5. Always stretch a warm muscle. Stretching a cold muscle is painful and not as effective.

Examples of some stretches will be found at the end of the chapter. There are many different types of stretches. One is usually not better than the other if done properly and when indicated. With this brief summary you should be able to judge exercises and decide when to use different types of stretching exercises.

ENERGY SOURCE DEVELOPMENT

A conditioning program prepares the body to perform a certain type and amount of work specific to a sport. In order to perform work, the body must have a resource of energy on which to rely. The development of the efficiency of the specific energy source of the body specific to the sport is the goal of a conditioning program.

There are three major types of energy sources in the body according to Mathews and Fox: ATP-PC, the lactic acid system, and the aerobic system [17]. The ATP-PC system takes the phosphocreatine that is stored in the muscles and breaks it down to creatine and a free phosphate. This causes a large amount of energy to be liberated. This energy is immediately available and is used directly to resynthesize ATP. In athletes the ATP-PC system is exemplified by the powerful, quick starts of sprinters, football players, high jumpers, and shot putters, and by similar feats that require only a few seconds to complete. This system is not dependent on a series of reactions nor on the oxygen we breathe and for this reason it represents the most rapid available source of ATP for use by the muscle.

The lactic acid system is another type of energy system that does not require oxygen. It takes place within the muscle cell and forms ATP by the incomplete breakdown of food to lactic acid. It uses only carbohydrates (glycogen and glucose) as its food fuel and produces relatively few ATP molecules. The food fuel enters the pathway in simple form as glucose but is stored in the muscle and liver as glycogen.

The aerobic system breaks down foodstuffs completely to CO_2 and H_2O in the presence of oxygen. This system utilizes all three foodstuffs (fats, proteins, carbohydrates) as fuels and yields a relatively large amount of ATP. The aerobic system is the more efficient system since lactic acid is not formed. Accumulations of high levels of lactic acid causes muscular fatigue. Even though the aerobic system is more efficient in producing ATP, it takes longer for its chemical reactions to take place. As a result, the lactic acid system is a very important energy source for activities that can be performed at a maximum rate for only two or three minutes. The aerobic energy system is predominantly used during long-term exercises that are performed at a submaximal rate since during such ativities there is ample time for the oxygen transport system to supply the muscle cells with enough oxygen to meet the ATP levels demanded by the exercise.

The length of time of intense activity in a sport will determine which energy system will predominate. For example, a football game will last three hours. If the intense activity of football lasted for the entire three hours the energy source would have to be aerobic. However, the average play from the line of scrimmage lasts only seven seconds, and is repeated many times during a game. The energy sources utilized in playing football would predominantly be the ATP-PC and the lactic acid system. A chart developed by Mathews and Fox gives examples of sports and energy systems that predominate [17].

From the previous sections, you realize that to increase muscular strength, the overload principle must be used by lifting greater amounts of weight. The same principle applies to the development of energy sources. Determine the energy source that is needed for the sport and develop it by repeating high intensity activities that will predominantly utilize that source of energy. This is illustrated in the interval training method. Interval training is a system of conditioning in which a series of repeated bouts of exercises alternated with periods of relief. The body is subjected to short but regularly repeated periods of work or stress interspersed with adequate periods of relief. Light or mild exercise usually constitutes this relief period. More work can be performed at a higher intensity since you have periods of relief. These relief periods delay the onset of fatigue by decreasing the amount of lactic acid accumulated.

Specifically, in regard to the development of the energy systems, intermittent work or the interval training system accomplishes the following:

1. It allows the ATP-PC system to be used over and over. This, in turn, provides an adequate stimulus for promoting an increase in the energy capacity of this system and aids in delaying the onset of fatigue by not delving so deeply into the lactic acid system [17].
2. With proper regulation of the duration and type of relief interval, the involvement of the lactic acid system will be maximal and thus improved.
3. By working long enough at a sufficient intensity and by improvement in the maximal attainable stroke volume, the aerobic system is developed.

There are many other types of training methods, but interval training is the most flexible, being able to adjust to whichever energy system is needed to be developed.

Another method to determine whether your workout is at a high enough intensity is to measure your pulse rate immediately after finishing the activity. This can be done by palpating the carotid pulse for ten seconds and multiplying by six. The target rate should be approximately two hundred minus your age. The target rate for periods of relief between repetition is approximately 160 minus your age. Between sets of exercise the target rate is even lower, approximately 140 minus age. Please refer to an exercise chart for exact figures [17].

Knowing these few physiological principles, the basis for an exercise program is available. Surprisingly, the amount of time practicing does not make as much of a difference as the intensity at which one works. The running of laps for a baseball player is good for off-season conditioning, but once the preseason workout begins, sprinting would be much more beneficial.

CONDITIONING AND INJURIES

With the better conditioned athlete, injuries should be decreased and performance should be increased due to the developed strength and stamina. The injured athlete has usually performed a stressful activity his or her body was not capable of withstanding. The adage of too much, too soon, or too fast usually can be applied. This is illustrated by the example of the Little League athlete who has "thrown out" his or her arm by their early teens. That individual tried to pitch several 6-inning games in one week over several seasons, not taking into account the number or type of pitches thrown. Children at a young age are not strong enough to withstand this amount of stress and injuries will result. If the athlete had been limited to the number of pitches thrown in one week and had been placed on a proper conditioning program, then his or her body would be able to adapt to the stress, and injuries of this nature would be avoided.

Physical adaptation of ligaments, tendons, and bone occurs when the body is placed in a stress situation for a period of time. Muscles and ligaments will thicken and adapt to stress, as well [9, 22]. Bones will increase the diameter of their cortical layer [26]. Obviously, a conditioning program provides a time during which these structures will adapt to the stress of a new activity. This will help to decrease the number of injuries and increase the work capabilities of an individual. A conditioning program should also increase the performance of the athlete. Strength and flexibility are not related to motor skills, but they have been shown to improve the potential abilities of an athlete when they are developed [4, 7, 18, 29]. There are some physical and motor abilties that are nondevelopmental and will affect the maximum athletic abilities of an individual. Skill levels are increased through training specific techniques of the sport. Skill drills should be incorporated into the conditioning program but should be thought of as a distinct section of the conditioning program.

Conditioning exercises should be individualized for the athlete the same way the skills are specific to the sport. The athlete's age, height, weight, previous athletic activities, and skill level should be considered when planning a conditioning program [28]. Most youngsters do not perform one particular sport year round. This is all to the good, for it is impractical to have a program that is specific to one event for a small child. As the youngster gets older, he or she may develop a preference for one sport. Then the overall program may lean to developing the physical attributes necessary for that sport.

The conditioning program, as the sport activitiy itself, must be enjoyable. If it becomes too much work, the child should not be heavily coaxed to continue. There is a psychological aspect to the conditioning program that you often do not consider when advising someone participating in sports. The era of the 14-year-old athlete not wanting to participate in sports because of high pressure and overexposure earlier in his career seems to be coming to an end. Remember to keep the "fun" aspect of any conditioning or athletic activity as a priority.

People involved with teaching sports skills to children should take time to develop a good conditioning program for them as well. Teaching a youngster how he can condition his body is something he can use for the rest of his life.

FLEXIBILITY SCREENING EXAMINATION AND EXERCISES

THOMAS TEST

This exam will help to determine the amount of anterior hip tightness of the athlete. This is typically found in individuals who have increased lumbar lordosis. The hip flexors act as an anchor holding the pelvis in an anteriorly rotated position, forcing the lumbar spine to become lordotic. By specifically stretching the structures on the anterior hip, without allowing any lordosis, it will enable a posterior pelvic tilt to be performed while standing.

To administer the test, have the patient lie supine with both knees held to the chest with hands. Do not allow the pelvis to rock up off the table. The examiner stands to the side of the athlete and palpates with the thumb of the hand most proximal to the athlete's head for the anterior superior iliac spine. The thumb is held on the anterior superior iliac spine for the entire exam. The other hand helps to lower the leg closest to the examiner while the patient continues to hold the other leg to his or her chest. When the examiner feels the movement of the anterior superior iliac spine inferiorly, a measurement is taken of the angle between the leg and the trunk of the patient. Both legs should be measured in case of a discrepancy. Normally the leg should be able to be lowered to the table without movement of the pelvis.

SUPINE STRAIGHT LEG RAISES

This examination tests for the relative tightness of the hamstrings. If done with the ankle held with maximal dorsiflexion, measurement will be of the flexibility of the entire posterior structures of the leg. A 90 degree angle between the leg and floor is an initial goal for any athlete. Some sports necessitate more flexibility of these structures to compete.

The test is administered with the athlete lying supine and the examiner by his or her side. One leg is slowly lifted off the table until the patient asks to stop movement. Position of the angle is noted. Careful consideration is given to ensure the knee remains in full extension. Measurement is taken of the angle between the trunk and long axis of the leg. Axis of the measurement is approximately the greater trochanter. Both legs are measured to check for discrepancies.

SUPINE DORSIFLEXION

This examination will determine the relative amount of flexibility of the plantar flexors, sometimes known as the "heel cords." The examiner stands at the bottom of the table while the athlete is supine with heels hanging slightly off the edge of table. The examiner supinates the foot to try and remove as much subtalar motion as possible, and gently presses the ankle into dorsiflexion. Measurement is taken by determining the angle between the imaginary line formed by the head of the fibula and the lateral malleolus and inferior border of the calcaneous. Measurements range approximately from 0 degrees of dorsiflexion (90 degrees) to 20 degrees of dorsiflexion. Average flexibility is between 10–15 degrees. Again careful consideration is taken to have the knee remain in full extension.

SUPINE SHOULDER FLEXION

This examination is to determine the relative amount of flexibility of the anterior structures of the shoulder joint. Tightness (flex) is sometimes found with athletes having posture difficulty (forward kyphosis, increased lordosis), sore elbows from tennis or baseball injuries, and inability to have a smooth throwing motion due to decreased shoulder flexibility. The test is administered with the athlete supine with hands at the side. The examiner passively moves the shoulder into flexion as far as possible without any resistance from tight structures. Once resistance is met, measurement is taken between long axis of trunk and arm with the axis of measurement approximately at the shoulder joint. Do not allow the athlete to arch his back while performing the test. Ideal range of motion is 180 degrees. Anything less is not pathological but continued stretch should be attempted to have full range of motion.

STANDING TOE TOUCH

This will provide a combined measure of the flexibility of the low back, hamstrings, and plantar flexors. By comparing straight leg raises with this measurement, the relative tightness of the hamstrings can be determined. Subjective observation will be a large factor in determining low back flexibility.

To administer the examination, the athlete stands and curls over to attempt to touch the floor and/or lean as far forward as possible. The examiner is standing in a position for a lateral view. Distance measurement is taken from tips of fingers to the floor with a tape measure and recorded in centimeters. The examiner will notice relative flexibility of upper back to lower back to hamstrings, which is contributing most to the athlete's ability to reach down to the floor. Determination is made and appropriate stretching flexibility exercises are issued. Scoliosis ribhump should also be examined from posterior view while patient is in this position.

NECK RANGE OF MOTION

Full neck range of motion and exceptional strength of neck musculature is essential to participation in some sports such as soccer and football. This will help to decrease the chance of injury to the cervical spine. The cervical spine has six basic movements and many of these combine to perform the spine's functional movements. Essentially these exercises will have the athlete actively move through the entire range of motion without any external forces applied. The first movement is flexion. Have the athlete sit with back supported. The athlete bends his or her neck forward trying to touch chin to chest. Measurement is taken from a lateral view, using the alignment of the trunk and the ear with the axis approximately through the cervical spine.

Extension of the neck is the second movement. The athlete bends his or her neck back as far as they can as if trying to see far above and behind them. Do not allow the thoracic or lumbar spine to arch. It is measured the same as flexion.

The third and fourth movements are lateral flexion to the left and right. With the athlete sitting ask him or her to bend the neck to the side and try to touch ear to shoulder. Make sure the shoulders do not elevate or the trunk will laterally bend. Measurement is taken from an anterior or posterior view and has the alignment of the trunk and midline of skull with the axis at the cervical spines.

The fifth and sixth movements are rotation to the left and right. The athlete is asked to turn the head as far as he or she can to one side. Rotation of the trunk is prevented by having the athlete seated with the back flush against the chair. Measurement is taken from a superior view. Alignment is the midline, sagittal plane, and the sagittal plane of the skull once the end of range of motion is reached. Axis is the cervical spine superior view.

STRENGTHENING EXERCISES

Strengthening exercises are necessary in the overall conditioning program for the child playing sports. Gradual progression of difficulty should be incorporated as the player masters the exercise. Caution should be used when increasing the difficulty of the exercises. Too fast an increase in weight or making the exercise too difficult could lead to injury. Children have a tendency to try to lift heavy weights without regard to proper technique. All weight training exercises should be well supervised with a coach who is aware of the proper techniques and progression of difficulty of the exercises. Weight training can and should be done throughout the year. In season weight training maintains strength and reduces chance of injury. Lifting should not be done prior to competition due to fatigue of the muscles being exercised. Stretching exercises should always precede and follow weight training to prepare the muscle for work and maintain its flexibility. Weight training can be done three times per week in the off season and twice per week in season.

The following are suggestions for muscle strengthening exercises that could be incorporated into your conditioning program. Perform them slowly, rhythmically, and without pain.

Neck Isometrics

Stand with feet shoulder width apart. Place both hands on forehead and push head forward but do not allow any neck movement. Put hand on either side of head. Press one hand, then the other, not allowing any neck movement. Now place both hands behind head and pull head forward. Do not allow neck movement. Repeat each direction 5 times, holding for 5 seconds.

Bicep Curls

Stand, keeping your back straight, throughout the exercise. Begin with your arm straight, palms facing forward, with your elbows in at your side. Bend your elbow, curling the weight up, bringing your hands toward your shoulders. Pause, lower slowly, and repeat making sure you fully extend the elbow with each repetition.

Shoulder Abduction

Stand, keeping your back straight, throughout the exercise. With the weight in your hand, arm straight, palms facing your side, lift your arm out to the side to shoulder height. Pause and lower slowly.

Shoulder Flexion

Stand, keeping your back straight, throughout the exercise. With the weight in your hand, arm straight, palms facing your side, lift the arm forward to shoulder height, keeping the elbow straight. Pause and lower slowly.

Tricep Extension

Lie on your stomach with your arm out to the side at shoulder level and your elbow bent over the edge of the plinth. With the weight in your hand, straighten the elbow, pause, and lower slowly.

Horizontal Abduction

Lie on your stomach close to the edge of the plinth so your arm may hang down off the edge. With the weight in your hand, lift your arm out to the side to shoulder level keeping your elbow straight. Pause and lower slowly.

Internal/External Rotation

Lie on your stomach so your arm is out to the side at shoulder level and your elbow is bent over the edge. With the weight in your hand, move your hand forward and then bend. Keep your elbow bent and in the same position on the plinth.

Horizontal Adduction

Lie on your back with your arm straight out in front of you at shoulder level. Lower the weights to the side, to the floor, and then return the weights to the starting position.

Straight Leg Raising

Longsitting position supported on elbows. One knee is bent and the other is straight with weight attached on the ankle or foot. Tighten your thigh muscle, keep your leg straight and your foot flexed up as you slowly lift it 12 to 18 inches off the floor. Hold, lower, relax, and repeat. Do not let your knee bend as you lift or lower the weight.

Hamstring Exercises

Standing, leaning over a table, with weight attached to one foot. Bend your knee, with weight attached to the foot, as far as you can. Pause, lower, relax, repeat.

Heel Walking

Lift your toes off the floor and walk on your heels. Keep your toes turned up and in. Walk for 45 feet and repeat 3 times.

Heel Raises

Stand with your toes slightly in (pigeon toed). Place front part of your foot on a 2 x 4. Rise up on your toes and lift your heels off the floor, pause, lower, and relax. This may be done while wearing a weighted vest or with weights on the shoulders.

Unilateral Balance

Stand on one foot with the other foot placed behind your knee. Place your hands on your hips. Balance for 60 seconds. When you can balance with your eyes open try repeating the same exercise with eyes closed.

Posterior Pelvic Tilt

Lie on your back with arms at side, hips and knees bent, and feet flat on the floor. Tighten your stomach muscles as you flatten your low back into the floor. Learn to do this with your knees straight also. Hold for 5 seconds, relax, and repeat 5 times.

Partial Situps

Lie on your back with your hands behind head and knees bent, feet unsupported. Perform a pelvic tilt. Place your chin on your chest and then raise your head and shoulders slowly from the mat. Sit half-way. Hold for 5 seconds, lower slowly, and repeat.

Both Knees to Chest–Lumbar Fascia Stretch

Lie on your back and bring both your knees to your chest. Grasp both knees with your hands; squeeze to chest. Do not rock pelvis off the floor. Feel stretch in low back. Hold for 10 seconds, relax, and repeat 5 times.

Lunge

Place hands on the floor with one leg straight behind you and the other knee bent closely under your chest. Keep your back leg straight and slowly lower your hips toward the floor. Feel stretch on front of hip with leg extended. Hold for 10 seconds, repeat 5 times.

Modified PNF–Yoga Butterfly

Sit "Indian" style with the soles of your feet together. Grab your ankles, and pull your feet as close to the hips as possible. Lower your knees toward the floor as far as you can. Give resistance with your elbows as you squeeze your knees together not allowing any leg movement. Hold for 5 seconds, relax, and again try to lower the knees toward the floor. Repeat 5 to 10 times.

Longsitting Toe Touch

Sit with your legs in front of you with knees straight and feet flexed toward face. Keeping your back straight, lean forward. Feel stretch on back legs. Hold for 5 to 10 seconds and repeat 5 times.

Modified PNF–Supine Hamstring Stretch

Lie on your back and lift one leg up off the ground as far as you can with your knee straight and ankle flexed toward face. Have partner hold leg as you press down for 5 seconds into his or her shoulder. Relax. Now lift leg away from shoulder of partner, keeping knee straight and ankle flexed. Partner should readjust to new position of leg. Now repeat pushing down into shoulder. Repeat procedure 5 times to each leg. Stretch should be felt in back of leg.

Side-Lying Quad Stretch

Lie on your left side, hold left knee to chest. Hold right ankle with right hand, extending hip and pull heel toward your seat. Hold as you tense quadricep muscle for a count of 5. Relax then extend hip further back and pull foot towards seat. Repeat 5 to 10 times. Roll over onto right side and repeat stretch to left leg.

Calf Stretch

Stand about two feet from partner with your feet shoulder width apart, toeing in slightly, with ankles slightly inverted. Keeping your body straight, lean into partner. Keep heels on the ground. If your heels come up, move closer to the partner. If you do not feel a stretch along your heelcords move your feet further away from your partner. Hold for 10 to 15 seconds. Repeat 3 to 5 times.

Trunk Stretch

Stand with feet shoulder width apart and arms extended above head. Bend forward, backwards, and side to side. Hold each position 5 seconds. Repeat 5 times.

Neck Stretches

Bend neck forward, back, side to side, and turn head to left and toward right. Again hold each position for 5 seconds and repeat 5 times.

REFERENCES

1. Astrand, P., and Rodahl, K.   *Textbook of Work Physiology* (2nd ed.). New York: McGraw-Hill 1977. P. 403.
2. Bennet, R.   Principles of Therapeutic Exercise. In S. Licht (Ed.), *Therapeutic Exercise* (2nd ed.). Baltimore: Waverly Press, 1965.
3. Brunnstrom, S.   *Clinical Kinesiology.* (3rd ed.), Philadelphia: Davis, 1972.
4. Campbell, R. L.   Effects of supplemental weight training on the physical fitness of athletic squads. *Res. Q. Am. Assoc. Health Phys. Ed.* 33:343, 1962.
5. Clarke, H. H.   *Muscular Strength and Endurance in Man.* Englewood Cliffs, N.J.: Prentice-Hall, 1966. See Chapter 4.
6. Cureton, T. K.   Flexibility as an aspect of physical fitness. *Res. Q. Am. Assoc. Health Phys. Educ.* 12:384, 1941.
7. Davis, J. F.   The effect of weight training on speed of swimming. *Phys. Ed.* 12:28, 1955.

8. Dickinson, R. V. The specificity of flexibility. *Res. Q. Am. Assoc. Health Phys. Educ.* 39:792, 1967.
9. Guyton, A. *Textbook of Medical Physiology* (5th ed.). Philadelphia: Saunders, 1976.
10. Hellebrant, F. A., and Houtz, S. J. Mechanisms of muscles training in man: Experimental demonstration of the overload principle. *Phy. Ther. Rev.* 36:371, 1956.
11. Hupprich, F., and Sigerseth, P. The specificity of flexibility in girls. *Res. Q. Am. Assoc. Health Phys. Educ.* 21:25, 1950.
12. Kabat, H. Proprioceptive facilitation in therapeutic exercise. In Sidney Licht (Ed.), *Principle of Therapeutic Exercise* (2nd ed.). Baltimore: Waverly Press, 1969.
13. Kendall, H., and Kendall, F. Normal flexibility according to age groups. *J. Bone Joint Surg. [AM.]* 39:424, 1948.
14. Knott, M., and Voss, D. *Proprioceptive Neuromuscular Facilitation—Patterns and Techniques* (2nd ed.). New York: Harper & Row, 1968.
15. Leighton, J. Flexibility characteristics of males ten to eighteen years of age. *J. Assoc. Phys. Ment. Rehab.* 10:494, 1956.
16. Leighton, J., et al. A study on the effectiveness of 10 different methods of progressive resistance exercise on the development of strength, flexibility, girth and body weight. *J. Assoc. Phys. Ment. Rehab.* 21:78, 1967.
17. Mathews, D. K., and Fox, E. L.: *The Physiological Basis of Physical Education and Athletics* (2nd ed.). Philadelphia: Saunders, 1976.
18. Meadows, P. E. The Effect of Isotonic and Isometric Muscle Contraction Training on Speed, Force, and Strength. University of Illinois Ph.D. Dissertation, 1959.
19. Micheli, L. J., et al. Assessment of lower extremity stress fractures in sports. *Med. Sci. Sports* 11:84, 1979.
20. Moore, M. L. The measurement of joint motion. *Phy. Ther. Rev.*, 24:195, 1949.
21. Northwestern University—Special Therapeutic Exercise Program, July 25, 1966–August 19, 1966. Proceedings: An exploratory and analytical survey of therapeutic exercise. *Am. J. Phy. Med.* 46(1), 1967.
22. Noyles, F. R., et al. Biomechanics of ligament failure. *J. Bone Joint Surg. [AM.]* 56:1406, 1974.
23. Personal Communication. Cybex: A Division of Lumex Inc. Sportsmedicine Department, 100 Spence Street, Bay Shore, NY 11706.
24. Personal Communication. Nautilus Sports/Medical Ind., P.O. Box 1783, DeLand, FL 32720.
25. Personal Communication. Universal Viking Fitness Corp., 43 Polk Avenue, Hempstead, NY 11550.
26. Salter, R. B. *Textbook of Disorders and Injuries of the Musculoskeletal System.* Baltimore: Williams & Wilkins, 1970.
27. Saltin, B. Metabolic fundamentals in exercise. *Med. Sci. Sports* 5:137, 1973.
28. Smith, R. J. Relationships Between Gross and Relative Strength and the Maturity, Physique Type, Body Size, and Motor Ability Elements of Boys Nine, Twelve, Fifteen and Seventeen Years of Age. University of Oregon Ph.D. Dissertation, 1968.
29. Thompson, C. W., and Martin, E. T. Weight training and baseball throwing speed. *J. Assoc. Phy. Mental Rehab.* 19:194, 1965.

Index